Redefining Resilience

Confronting Systemic Omissions and Impacts in Educational Policy

Shaheen Shariff
General Editor

Vol. 4

The Confronting Systemic Omissions and Impacts in Educational Policy series is part of the Peter Lang Education list.

Every volume is peer reviewed and meets the highest quality standards for content and production.

PETER LANG
New York · Berlin · Bruxelles · Chennai · Lausanne · Oxford

Redefining Resilience

Overcoming Social Challenges During and After COVID-19

Shaheen Shariff, Christopher Dietzel,
Safia Amiry, and Safeera Jaffer (eds.)

PETER LANG
New York · Berlin · Bruxelles · Chennai · Lausanne · Oxford

Bibliographic information published by the Deutsche Nationalbibliothek
The Deutsche Nationalbibliothek lists this publication in the Deutsche Nationalbibliografie; detailed bibliographic data are available on the Internet at https://dnb.dnb.de.

Library of Congress Cataloging-in-Publication Data
Names: Dietzel, Christopher, 1989- editor | Amiry, Safia, 1989- editor | Jaffer, Safeera, 1996- editor
Title: Redefining resilience: overcoming social challenges during and after COVID-19 / [edited by] Shaheen Shariff, Christopher Dietzel, Safia Amiry, Safeera Jaffer.
Identifiers: LCCN 2026010987 (print) | LCCN 2026010988 (ebook) | ISBN 9783034358644 paperback | ISBN 9783034358866 pdf | ISBN 9783034358873 epub
Subjects: LCSH: COVID-19 Pandemic, 2020-2023--Social aspects | COVID-19 Pandemic, 2020-2023--Influence | Students--Mental health
Classification: LCC RA644.C67 R395 2026 (print) | LCC RA644.C67 (ebook)
LC record available at https://lccn.loc.gov/2026010987
LC ebook record available at https://lccn.loc.gov/2026010988

This work was supported by iMPACTS: Collaborations to Address Sexual Violence on Campus; Social Sciences and Humanities Research Council of Canada Partnership Grant Number: 895-2016-1026, Project Director, Shaheen Shariff, Distinguished James McGill Professor Emerita, McGill University.

Artwork by Professor Emerita Shaheen Shariff
Cover design by Alyssa Jetha

ISSN 2834-6939
ISBN 978-3-0343-5864-4 (Print)
ISBN 978-3-0343-5886-6 (ePDF)
ISBN 978-3-0343-5887-3 (ePUB)
DOI 10.3726/b22922

Published by Peter Lang Publishing Inc., New York, USA

info@peterlang.com

This publication has been peer reviewed.

www.peterlang.com

Contact for General Product Safety Regulation (GPSR): gpsr@peterlang.com

Dedication from Shaheen Shariff, Distinguished James McGill Professor Emerita

For my incredible team of graduate and post-graduate research associates and research assistants. I know that each of you will succeed in your careers because of your work ethic, insight, and dedication.

Dedication from Christopher Dietzel, PhD

To the many individuals and communities who have felt the lasting impacts of the COVID-19 pandemic.

Dedication from Safia Amiry

To all whose experiences of inequality remind us that the struggle for justice and equity is both personal and collective.

Dedication from Safeera Jaffer

To all the people who experience the ongoing COVID-19 pandemic as intricately tied to other systems of oppression. While these forces are connected, so too is liberation.

CONTENTS

ACKNOWLEDGEMENT OF FUNDING

This work was supported by *iMPACTS: Collaborations to Address Sexual Violence on Campus*; Social Sciences and Humanities Research Council (SSHRC) of Canada Partnership Grant Number: 895-2016-1026, Project Director: Shaheen Shariff, Distinguished James McGill Professor Emerita, McGill University.

TABLES

PREFACE BY THE EDITORS

As the impacts of the COVID-19 pandemic have been felt globally, the social dimensions of these effects have also been intense, unequal and significant (Altmejd et al., 2023; Schweiger, 2023; Thomas et al., 2023). It is crucial to recognize the social consequences of the pandemic, which have influenced education, employment, public perceptions and well-being. For example, in the field of education, research shows that the pandemic has substantially affected global experiences of teaching and learning, including from K–12 to higher education (Al Mazrooei et al., 2023; Ryan, 2023).

Importantly, as people adapted to changing circumstances emerging from the pandemic, the social factors have also changed over time. As we move forward and learn to live with the COVID-19 virus, it is important to examine the social aspects of the COVID-19 pandemic, both past and present. These short- and long-term consequences provide the basis for this edited volume, which explores the social impacts of the pandemic on people and their everyday lives. This edited collection brings together research from multiple countries, mainly focusing on Canada and the United Kingdom. The overarching goal of this edited book is to examine the social experiences of people during the pandemic, how they responded, the implications for broader society, and what we can learn moving forward. Each of the chapters highlights valuable findings that have implications for healthcare, education and social policy and the intricate connections between them.

The concept of social justice allows us to scrutinize the uneven and disproportionate impacts of the COVID-19 pandemic on diverse populations. Due to the systemic forces of privilege and oppression within and beyond healthcare, the ramifications of the pandemic have been highly inequitable. Research conducted since 2020 has demonstrated how the individual and collective social positions of historically marginalized populations have faced larger barriers and experienced greater negative consequences related to COVID-19 (Cox, 2020; Craig, 2023; Silva & Smith, 2020). Because of these multiple and interlocking forces, marginalized groups have faced increased challenges from the health and social dimensions of the pandemic – and with lasting effects. Considering the geographical focus of this collection, recent studies have shown how various populations in Canada (see Datta Gupta et al., 2022; Singh Kelsall et al., 2023) and the United Kingdom (see Basch et al., 2022; Lemyre & Messina, 2023) have navigated the intricacies of the COVID-19 pandemic amongst their own social, political and economic contexts. As such, taking a social justice approach allows us to explore and understand the often-overlooked social consequences of a virus.

As demonstrated in this collection, the social dimensions of the pandemic have not only affected people's physical and mental health, but also people's everyday social interactions in schools, workplaces and other spaces. These social issues go beyond individual impacts and extend to families, colleagues and communities. Through the lens of social justice, we can examine the multiplicity of challenges exacerbated by the pandemic and scrutinize how factors such as class, age, race, employment, caste, dis/ability, nationality and technological access, among others, can drastically influence people's social experiences.

This collection, which focuses on education and employment sectors, examines social issues posed by the pandemic, emphasizing how public health interventions and societal behaviours influenced the collective experience. This approach lays the groundwork for a better understanding of the pandemic's widespread impacts. The collection begins by looking at the education sector, which progresses from K–12 to post-secondary education and highlights the considerable changes in learning environments while also demonstrating the broader societal ramifications of these shifts. This collection concludes with a study of the pandemic's economic consequences, analysing how the crisis changed work, labour dynamics and financial institutions across numerous sectors. By exploring these issues, the collection considers the pandemic's long-term effects and underscores the need for systemic changes and innovative recovery strategies.

Chapter 1 – The Impact of the COVID-19 Pandemic on French Immersion Students and Families

This chapter by Roksana Dobrin-De Grace, Elizabeth Kay-Raining Bird, Diana Burchell, Kathleen Hipfner-Boucher and Xi Chen explores the experiences of French Immersion (FI) students and their families during online learning amid the COVID-19 pandemic. Although parents acknowledged certain advantages, such as enhanced technology skills and easier access to resources, many were dissatisfied with the decreased exposure to spoken French – a crucial component of FI education that was challenging to maintain outside of the classroom. The study also draws attention to the additional difficulties experienced by lower-income families and children with special education needs (SEN). School-provided resources were often insufficient to support French literacy, leaving lower-income families struggling to balance work and their children's education. On the other hand, some higher-income families were able to leave their jobs to focus on their children's education and employ private tutors to improve their children's French language skills. The chapter highlights the importance of providing additional support for FI students, particularly those from disadvantaged communities and those with SEN, so that they have equitable access to learning and academic performance.

Chapter 2 – The Ripple Effect: Post-secondary Students, Systemic Inequity and the COVID-19 Pandemic

In this chapter, Serenity Friskie and Sunny Manhas investigate the heightened effects of the COVID-19 pandemic on marginalized post-secondary students in British Columbia, particularly those with intersecting identities related to race, gender and socioeconomic status. The findings show how the pandemic exacerbated existing issues such as financial insecurity, mental health difficulties and encounters with racism and gender-based violence. These experiences demonstrate that the challenges faced by these students are not simply new impediments but rather an increased reflection of long-standing systemic inequalities that have perpetually affected their educational paths. The chapter emphasizes the urgent need for post-secondary institutions to implement anti-racism policies and actively participate in the Truth and Reconciliation Commission's 94 Calls to Action. Prioritising these measures allows schools to create equitable educational environments that fully recognize and address the different needs of all students. This strategy not only promotes diversity but also empowers marginalized voices, creating a supportive environment where every student has the opportunity to thrive.

Chapter 3 – Between the Rock and the Hard Place: Exploring the Effects of COVID-19 on One Student's Mental Well-Being in England Using the Auto-Hermeneutic Approach

Zineb Boudiba provides a personal account of being a PhD student in the UK during the COVID-19 pandemic to critically examine the social struggles faced by international students at this time. Through an auto-hermeneutic approach and a narrative review, Boudiba reflects on the profound psychological and social challenges experienced during this period, including isolation, disconnection from loved ones and uncertainty related to the pandemic. A key contribution of the chapter is its innovative application of auto-hermeneutics to explore social struggles in a health context, marking the first time this method has been used to assess the impact of COVID-19 on international students. Boudiba emphasizes the importance of addressing the social and emotional needs of international students during global crises, calling for more attention to their unique challenges.

Chapter 4 – The Need to Reconsider the Occupational Rights of Low-Wage Essential Workers Post-Pandemic

In the book's final chapter, Steven Kupidy and Lynn Shaw investigate the shift from non-essential to essential that low-wage workers experienced during the COVID-19 pandemic. By focusing on this transition in work identity, Kupidy and Shaw analyse workers' sense of belonging and well-being and uncover significant challenges that low-wage workers faced as they became regarded as "essential." The authors advocate for comprehensive government policies to alleviate the problems affecting essential workers and to provide ongoing support. They also call for a broader definition of essential work so that it considers not only the nature of work but also workers' rights and protections. Overall, this chapter emphasizes the importance of policy reforms, better hiring practices and increased protections that promote the safety, dignity and well-being of essential workers, thereby proposing systematic changes that can better support these individuals whose employment is often precarious.

References

Al Mazrooei, A. K., Hatem Almaki, S., Gunda, M., Alnoor, A., & Manji Sulaiman, S. (2023). A systematic review of K-12 education responses to emergency remote teaching during the COVID-19 pandemic. *International Review of Education: Journal of Lifelong Learning, 68*(6), 811–841. https://doi.org/10.1007/s11159-023-09986-w.

Altmejd, A., Östergren, O., Björkegren, E., & Persson, T. (2023). Inequality and COVID-19 in Sweden: Relative risks of nine bad life events, by four social gradients, in pandemic vs. prepandemic years. *Proceedings of the National Academy of Sciences, 120*(46). https://doi.org/10.1073/pnas.2303640120.

Basch, C., Nielsen, J., Rabbani, M., Alhuzali, H., Zhang, T., & Ananiadou, S. (2022). Emotions and topics expressed on Twitter during the COVID-19 pandemic in the United Kingdom: Comparative geolocation and text mining analysis. *Journal of Medical Internet Research, 24*(10), Article e40323. https://doi.org/10.2196/40323.

Cox, C. (2020). Older adults and Covid 19: Social justice, disparities, and social work practice. *Journal of Gerontological Social Work, 63*(6), 611–624. https://doi.org/10.1080/01634372.2020.1808141.

Craig, G. (ed.). (2023). *Social Justice in a Turbulent Era*. Edward Elgar Publishing. https://doi.org/10.4337/9781803926155.

Datta Gupta, S., Engler-Stringer, R., Ruetz, A., & McKenna, M. L. (2022). School food programming across Canada during the COVID 19 pandemic: Program reach and modalities. *Journal of Hunger & Environmental Nutrition, 18*(3), 343–355. https://doi.org/10.1080/19320248.2022.2105185.

Lemyre, A., & Messina, J. P. (2023). Greenspace use during the COVID-19 pandemic: A longitudinal population mobility study in the United Kingdom. *Environmental Research, 239*, Article 117360. https://doi.org/10.1016/j.envres.2023.117360.

Ryan, J. M. (ed.). (2023). *Pandemic pedagogies: Teaching and learning during the COVID-19 pandemic*. Routledge. https://doi.org/10.4324/9781003324096.

Schweiger, G. (ed.). (2023). *The Global and Social Consequences of the COVID-19 Pandemic*. Springer. https://doi.org/10.1007/978-3-030-97982-9.

Silva, D. S., & Smith, M. J. (2020). Social distancing, social justice, and risk during the COVID-19 pandemic. *Canadian Journal of Public Health, 111*(4), 459–461. https://doi.org/10.17269/s41997-020-00354-x.

Singh Kelsall, T., DeBeck, K., Grant, C., Gorbach, P., Milloy, M.-J., & Hayashi, K. (2023). Food insecurity during the COVID-19 pandemic who use drugs in Vancouver, Canada. *Public Health Nutrition, 26*(9), 1878–1886. https://doi.org/10.1017/S1368980023001234.

Thomas, M. E., Henderson, L. M., & Horton, H. D. (2023). *Race, Ethnicity, and the COVID-19 Pandemic*. University of Cincinnati Press. https://muse.jhu.edu/book/123562.

· 1 ·

THE IMPACT OF THE COVID-19 PANDEMIC ON FRENCH IMMERSION STUDENTS AND FAMILIES

Roksana Dobrin-De Grace, Elizabeth Kay-Raining Bird, Diana Burchell, Kathleen Hipfner-Boucher and Xi Chen

This chapter describes the early experiences of online learning during the COVID-19 pandemic among French Immersion (FI) students and their families. Previous research has shown that Canadian children and their families faced numerous logistical, educational and emotional challenges with virtual learning. However, much less is known about the impact of the pandemic on early elementary FI students, specifically those from lower-income backgrounds in Toronto, Ontario. In this study, we conducted semi-structured interviews with eight parents from diverse socio-economic backgrounds, mostly from English-speaking households. The findings revealed that FI parents were generally unsatisfied and frustrated with guiding and assisting their children through their virtual learning experiences. Parents expressed concern regarding their children's reduced exposure to spoken French from teachers and peers as a consequence of not being in an in-person classroom, as well as the costs and difficulty of obtaining French resources. Parents spoke of other issues, such as their children's declining mental health, difficulties communicating with the school regarding their children's progress, and the strain of juggling work and the need to support their children's virtual learning despite not speaking French themselves. These challenges, particularly securing French language assistance and providing schoolwork support at home, were accentuated in lower-income families. Due to decreased French exposure during lockdown, FI students can benefit from increased French language input and access to French resources, especially those in under-served schools and communities. Importantly, our findings highlight the need to support families with students who have special education needs in FI as a route to increasing diversity in the FI programme.

The COVID-19 pandemic brought unprecedented educational challenges for students, teachers and families, with stay-at-home orders forcing many school boards worldwide to move to online learning. Many countries, including Canada, adopted exclusively virtual or hybrid learning settings during the peak periods of the pandemic (Schleicher, 2020). Early in the pandemic, in the spring semester of 2020, much of students' learning was conducted online asynchronously, which meant that teachers recorded their lessons and provided work for students to watch and complete independently. In late 2020, Ontario teachers pivoted their online practice to teach synchronously (i.e. in real time) online for most of the school day. In 2021, parents could choose whether to keep their children in virtual synchronous learning or opt for in-person school. Currently, Ontario schools are back to in-person instruction (Government of Ontario, 2022).

Since stay-at-home orders caused considerable disruption to regular schooling in 2020, it is vital to understand the educational challenges that students and families faced during this year. Importantly, since the long-term effects of the COVID-19 pandemic remain uncertain and other pandemics may occur, understanding how families have navigated these schooling modifications academically and psychologically can help prepare us for future challenges.

Although several studies have examined the impact of the pandemic on online schooling experiences more broadly (e.g. Domina et al., 2021; Garbe et al., 2020; Kaffenberger, 2021; Kuhfeld et al., 2020), few studies have investigated its impact on French Immersion (FI) students in Canada, particularly those with special education needs (SEN) or who come from a lower socio-economic status (SES). The present study seeks to address the gap in the literature by investigating the impact of the COVID-19 pandemic on the experiences of FI families from diverse backgrounds in Toronto, Ontario.

Overview of the French Immersion Programme in Canada

The purpose of the FI programme in Canada is to support English–French bilingualism by providing English-speaking Canadians access to French-language instruction in public schools (Lazaruk, 2007). Presently, there are no restrictions on who can enrol, and the programme is open to families from diverse language backgrounds, although FI classrooms are not available in all public schools or communities. FI is selectively offered in a small number of schools (often concentrated in more wealthy neighbourhoods), and children could attend if they live close to the school or if they join a lottery (Yoon et al., 2022). The lottery process changes with each school board, but generally, the school board advertises the FI programme both in school and in the community, and invites parents to either enrol directly if they live in the catchment area or to sign their child up for the lottery system in which students are randomly selected to participate in the programme. While some school boards have started to reserve a certain proportion of spots for under-represented students in the lottery, this is not a universal practice and has also come with issues. For example, in the Toronto District School Board (TDSB), an error in this process further excluded marginalized students (Teotonio, 2023).

Since its inception in the 1960s, the Canadian FI programme has been highly successful. Benefits of the programme for FI students include expanded job opportunities (Lazaruk, 2007), higher engagement in school (Sinay, 2010), a better appreciation of different cultures and languages (Lazaruk, 2007), and cognitive gains such as mental flexibility and creative thinking skills (Lazaruk, 2007) compared to students in the regular English stream. Throughout the programme, typically developing children in FI (those without a confirmed diagnosis of neurodiversity or a learning disability) perform equivalently or better than their peers in English programmes (Lindholm-Leary & Genesee, 2014). In terms of language, these FI students obtain similar levels of English proficiency as their English-stream peers once English language classes are introduced, usually by third grade. While FI students do not obtain native-like proficiency, they score considerably higher on French language and literacy skills compared to students who take French as a second language within the English programmes (Lindholm-Leary & Genesee, 2014).

Diversity in the French Immersion Programme

The FI programme in Canada is becoming increasingly more diverse in terms of students' language background, ethnicity, SES, and ability (Egbo, 2009); however, inequality persists and there are some stark demographic differences between the English and the FI streams (Sinay et al., 2018). As an example, 26–31 % of the TDSB student body is white, compared to 48–50 % in its FI programme. While there is no simple explanation for why this occurs, it is possible that FI requires additional financial support to remain in the programme (e.g. tutors, extracurricular activities) that only higher SES families can afford, many of which are disproportionately white (Kunnas, 2019). Indeed, parents with higher incomes and a university education are more likely to enrol their children in FI, while fewer children with SEN attend FI than the TDSB as a whole (3.5 % compared to 14.9 %) (Sinay et al., 2018). Although these percentages may be different depending on the region or the province, the TDSB serves as an example of the stark discrepancies between the two streams.

Children with SEN in FI have also been shown to perform academically at similar or better levels than their SEN peers in English language programmes, and they develop French language and literacy skills (Genesee & Lindholm-Leary, 2021; Kay-Raining Bird et al., 2021).

It is important to note that there may be a self-selection effect in that children with SEN in FI may be more high-functioning than children with SEN in English-language programmes. The evidence cited also comes primarily from English-speaking provinces. Nevertheless, despite evidence that students with SEN in FI do not necessarily suffer academically in remaining in these programmes, FI programmes often lack sufficient special education support compared to English programmes. The services that are available to students with SEN (for example, individualized, one-on-one support such as reading assistance) are infrequently offered in French (Mady & Muhling, 2017; Wise, 2011).

For children with SEN who are struggling, this may lead parents to seek support (e.g. assessments or interventions) outside the school system (Selvachandran et al., 2022). However, because external support is costly, it is not always accessible. Consequently, parents, especially those with low incomes, may feel that their only option is to withdraw their children from FI to access the services their children need (Kay-Raining Bird et al., 2021). Taken together, students from racialized backgrounds, low SES backgrounds and with SEN are not proportionally reflected in the FI student population. This is largely due to the additional costs required to succeed in the programme and the lack of adequate support for students with SEN.

Challenges in French Immersion Programmes During the COVID-19 Pandemic

The COVID-19 pandemic presented numerous educational challenges. While school closures and online learning kept families safe from COVID-19, research has shown that we can expect significant delays in literacy and mathematics achievement for elementary school students worldwide as a result (Kaffenberger, 2021; Kuhfeld et al., 2020). In addition, the COVID-19 pandemic had exacerbated difficulties in accessing appropriate special education services for children with SEN generally and particularly in FI since many internal and external supports were temporarily unavailable (Asbury et al., 2021; Neece et al., 2020).

Research specifically examining FI programmes in Canada during the COVID-19 pandemic has been scarce. In one noteworthy qualitative study, Fontenelle-Tereshchuk (2021) interviewed parents of elementary English-stream and FI students during the early 2020 school lockdown in Alberta, Canada. Parents in both streams were generally dissatisfied with the state of online learning and found it unreasonable to expect elementary school children to work independently at home. As discussed previously, these parents also needed to provide considerable educational support to their children, along with their own work and home responsibilities. Parents of FI children specifically noted that when their children struggled to complete the assigned work, they could provide only minimal support due to their "weak" French skills, as most of the parents in the sample did not speak French (Fontenelle-Tereshchuk, 2021). For those parents who did speak French, the educational instruction was easier, although they felt a burden of responsibility for teaching their children the language (Fontenelle-Tereshchuk, 2021).

Similar sentiments were expressed by a group of parents interviewed in British Columbia (including some with children in FI) (MacDonald & Hill, 2022). The parents reported wanting to be active participants in their children's schooling, but they expressed concern that the work assigned by teachers required too much of parents' time and effort, especially as many worked from home and had to juggle the demands of both work and their children's schooling. The shift to virtual learning blurred the roles for many parents who felt that they acted as both the parent and the teacher to their children. Little was reported with regard to parents' experiences with FI specifically. Although somewhat dissimilar to our present study, which focuses on FI elementary school students, the authors also interviewed secondary school FI teachers on their experiences (MacDonald & Hill, 2022). The teachers expressed concern that the French homework they received during this period was clearly completed with the help of the parents, having little to no spelling and grammar mistakes and using complex verb tenses (MacDonald & Hill, 2022).

Present Study

While several studies have looked at the learning outcomes of students and the experiences of families and teachers during the COVID-19 pandemic generally, little is known about the impact of online learning on children in bilingual programmes such as FI, especially the impact on diverse FI students, including those from lower-income backgrounds and students with SEN. In addition, little is known about the experiences of families in the early FI programme in Toronto, Ontario, which serves a largely different demographic than Alberta and British Columbia (Fontenelle-Tereshchuk, 2021; MacDonald & Hill, 2022).

We sought to address these gaps in the literature by interviewing parents of children in early FI programmes (Grades 1–3) from diverse backgrounds in Toronto, Ontario, about their experiences during the pandemic. Our sample included families from low SES backgrounds and families whose children have SEN. The following research question guided our analysis: How did the shift to online learning during the COVID-19 pandemic impact the educational experiences of early FI families from diverse backgrounds?

Methods

This qualitative study explored the impact of the COVID-19 pandemic on the learning experiences of early FI students and their families in Toronto through semi-structured interviews with the parents. The participants were recruited through a larger SSHRC-funded study: the International Bilingual Education (IBE) Project, which examined FI children's language and literacy development across Ontario. We investigated children's and parents' experiences in both the early asynchronous stage of online learning during the spring semester in early 2020 and the later synchronous stage in the fall semester of 2020.

We asked parents what the benefits and challenges of online learning were during the COVID-19 pandemic; we then analysed these responses to see whether families' experiences varied as a function of SES or SEN. We used Braun and Clark's (2006) thematic analysis, a prevalent method used to identify and guide the analytical process of qualitative data.

Participants

Eight parents whose children were enrolled in a FI programme in four different primary public schools participated in this study. The participating parents were all mothers and resided in Toronto, Canada. All parents had at least one child in the early FI programme, with some having other children who were either older or younger in the FI programme or in the English stream. None of the interviewed parents was a fluent French speaker, although some had basic French knowledge.

Parents were recruited through the larger IBE Project, who had previously agreed to be contacted through the IBE Project for other studies. When contacting potential participants by email, we implemented both a general recruitment strategy (contacting all parents in the IBE Project) and a targeted recruitment strategy (contacting lower SES schools based on TDSB's Learning Opportunities Index[1], LOI; for more information, see Toronto District School Board, 2020). Recruitment lasted approximately two months and we aimed for diversity in recruiting in terms of family SES and number of children in the home with SEN. However, there were no specific inclusion or exclusion criteria. Participants were compensated with a $20 e-transfer upon completion of the interview.

Participants completed a demographic questionnaire created by the research team that provided indices of family and school SES and information about family make-up (Table 1.1). School SES was determined using the school board LOI. Family income was the proxy for family SES, classified as low (≤ $49,999; *n* = 4), middle ($50,000–$99,999; *n* = 3) or high (≥ $100,000; *n* = 1). Five families had children with SEN. Where known, details are provided about parents' specific work situations (if not specified, the information was not provided). A more detailed description of the participants' families can be found in Table 1.2.

Table 1.1: Demographic Information of the Participants (*n* = 8)

ID	School SES	Family SES	Parent Born in Canada	Adults in the Home	Children in the Home (#SEN in FI)
1MH1	Mid	High	Yes	2 parents	2 (1)
2MH1	Mid	High	No	2 parents	2 (1)
3HH0	High	High	Yes	2 parents	2 (0)
4LM2	Low	Mid	Yes	2 parents	3 (2)
5MM0	Mid	Mid	No	2 parents	2 (0)
6LL1	Low	Low	Yes	1 parent	1 (1)
7LL1	Low	Low	No	2 parents	4 (1)
8LL0	Low	Low	Yes	1 parent	1 (0)

Note: Participant identification consists of the participant number + school SES (L = low, M = Mid, H = high) + family SES (L = low, M = Mid, H = high) + # children with suspected or diagnosed SEN in the family who are in the FI programme. For example, 8LL0 = 8th parent, low school SES, low family SES, no children with SEN in FI.

1 The Learning Opportunities Index ranks TDSB schools based on measures of external challenges affecting student success, including school board census data.

Table 1.2: Parent and Child Descriptive Information

ID	Parent Information	Child Information
1MH1	Father worked full-time (hybrid). Mother worked full-time but left her job to help her children with school when the pandemic started.	Two children: twins. One, typically developing and doing well in FI (defined henceforth as not struggling academically in FI). The other had suspected learning problems and struggled in FI.
2MH1	Both parents had full-time jobs. Mother worked from home.	Two children. The older, typically developing and doing well in FI. The younger, suspected of learning/ emotional problems and in FI.
3HH0	Both parents had full-time jobs.	Two children. Both typically developing in FI and doing well.
4LM2	Father worked full-time outside the home and mother worked part-time but paused her work during online learning.	Three children. The oldest graduated high school in FI and did well. The second, diagnosed with a learning disability and anxiety disorder, transferred from FI to an English programme. The youngest, suspected of learning disability and in FI.
5MM0	Both parents had full-time jobs (hybrid).	Two children. Both typically developing in FI and doing well.
6LL1	Single-parent household. Worked full-time (from home during online learning).	One child. Typically developing with suspected socio-emotional issues in FI and doing well.
7LL1	Father worked full-time (outside the home). Mother stayed home with the children.	Four children. The oldest, non-verbal and in an English special education programme. The second, typically developing in FI and doing well. The third, suspected attention deficit and in FI. The youngest, not in school yet.
8LL0	Single-parent household. Mother worked full-time (from home during online learning).	One child. Typically developing in FI and doing well.

Interviews

Two trained graduate students (the first and second authors, trained by the third author, who has more expertise in qualitative research) conducted 90-minute online semi-structured interviews using Zoom. Participants were asked to take the call in a private, quiet area in their homes where their children would not overhear the interview. All interviews were conducted in English and audio recorded for later transcription and analysis. Participants were asked questions about their family's FI experiences, how schooling was modified in response to the COVID-19 pandemic, and the family's responses to those modifications. Participants were prompted to elaborate with follow-up questions if more details were required for a more comprehensive understanding.

The interview protocol was piloted with two parents and modified, mainly by adjusting the question order and making minor wording changes, to ensure it effectively elicited a dialogue pertinent to the research question. Since these interviews are part of a larger study, only responses to the questions directly related to COVID-19 pandemic experiences are reported in this chapter.

Analysis

The interviews were initially transcribed using Otter.ai, an online transcription programme. The second author trained a research assistant on standard transcription conventions (Dresing et al., 2015). The research assistant applied the Dresing et al. (2015) conventions to the transcripts, checked the transcripts while listening to the recorded interviews to correct errors, and anonymized identifying information.

The transcribed interviews were then analysed thematically using an iterative process (Braun & Clarke, 2006). The iterative process involved all authors reading the interviews; identifying components of the transcripts that inductively reflected important aspects of the participants' experiences; and creating themes, subthemes and codes by consensus through discussion. Demographic characteristics of the participants and their families were used to determine whether theme and subtheme expression varied across SES and the presence of child(ren) with SEN.

Results

Figure 1.1 presents the results of the thematic analysis. The results section is organized around two main themes: children's experiences and parents' experiences. Under each theme are the main subthemes. Under children's experiences, parents mainly discussed the benefits and difficulties of online learning. Under parents' experiences, parents spoke of the impact of virtual schooling on their own work, their role as teachers to their children, and the cost of acquiring extra support. In addition, most subthemes are further divided into the most discussed topics.

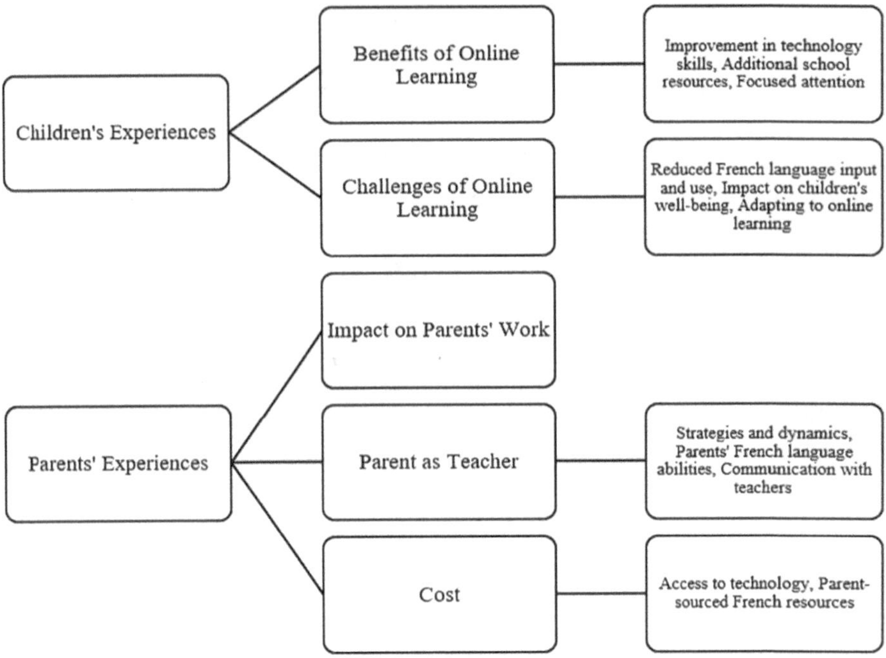

Figure 1.1: Themes and Subthemes.

Children's Experiences

Mothers talked about both the benefits and challenges of the COVID-19 schooling modifications for their children. The identified primary benefits of virtual schooling included children's improvement in technology skills, additional school resources and focused attention. Parents more often spoke of the challenges with online learning, including reduced French language input and use, the negative impact on children's well-being, particularly the increase in stress and anxiety, and the difficulty adapting to virtual schooling.

Benefits of Online Learning

Improvement in Technology Skills

All parents acknowledged that their children acquired new technological skills during the pandemic. While children needed considerable support at the beginning of the pandemic to learn to use the required technology (e.g. computers, tablets and web-based applications such as Zoom and Google Classroom), they felt their children became quite skilled at their use:

> But from a technology perspective, I think they're good. Like, now he can navigate everything like all this Google Classroom where he knows even better than I do now. Where his assignments [are]..., what to do and like, where to login and logout. (Parent 5MM0)

Additional School Resources

Parents reported that schools purchased temporary educational resources, which helped with online learning during the COVID-19 pandemic. As Parent 1MH1 said: "I think the one positive of all that was that the teachers had more access to money that allowed them to access different resources across the board for all the students in the class". Helpful resources included a website that offered French books of different levels, Raz Kids and Boukili, a French reading application. Parents expressed appreciation for these resources, saying they helped them support their children's French reading development and were fun to use.

Focused Attention

Some parents worked from home during the pandemic or were financially secure enough to reduce their working hours. These parents enjoyed being able to interact more frequently with their children during school lockdowns, such as Parent 4LM2: "I would say the biggest benefit, being able to have one-on-one time with my kid and being able to explain things to them. But again, not every family has that opportunity, right?" Parent 1MH1, who had a child with attention difficulties, suggested that asynchronous learning might be more beneficial for students who were able to focus and work independently.

Challenges with Online Learning

Reduced French Language Input and Use

Parents feared that their children's French language acquisition would be delayed. FI students do not typically obtain additional French language exposure by means of a French language speaker outside the classroom environment (Rehner & Mougeon, 2003). Based on their observations of children's lessons, many parents were concerned that the children were not being adequately exposed to French, especially early in the pandemic when all classes were asynchronous.

> How many months was it without [a word of] French, to try and learn the language when you are not conversing. … they're watching movies in French and we make sure they read … but it's not the same as when the teachers repeat the same sentences every day until they get it. I think that part could have definitely been organized much better. (Parent 2MH1)

Parents also reported that teachers would frequently revert to English during online lessons, perhaps because teachers found it difficult to adjust and maintain students' attention or adequately respond to students' variable French language abilities in a virtual context: "I'm assuming the teachers are frustrated because they're responding in English and they're not supporting … speaking in French and maintaining that consistency in French" (Parent 6LL1).

Many parents expressed concerns that their children had few opportunities to interact with teachers or peers in French. As Parent 4LM2 stated:

> The minimum requirement needs to be the teachers in front of the cameras talking to the kids. … I think they need the time with their teachers, they should be actually spending time talking to the rest of their class and having a bit of socialization through that as well.

As this parent implied, such interactions were important for more than their children's French development.

Some parents in our study expressed the view that the negative effects on French might be temporary, at least for younger children:

> I mean, the oral part they really lost out on, but I don't think for my kids anyway that that's been a huge loss. I think that just by keeping them going with the writing and the reading that they're back in the classroom now, thankfully, and that whatever was lost there will be picked up pretty quickly at their age. (Parent 1MH1)

It should be noted that parents who were less concerned about the long-term impacts were those with higher incomes and the ability to work more with their children at home.

Impact on Children's Well-Being

Parents frequently expressed concerns that their children did not enjoy online learning or that it negatively impacted their children's mental health, especially but not exclusively for those students who had known or suspected mental health challenges, such as anxiety, prior to the pandemic. Parent 6LL1, for example, reported that the disruption in her daughter's routine resulted in an attitude shift:

> I just feel her relationship with education has changed. This was a kid who I had no problem rising at 6:50 AM every morning to go to daycare drop off, knowing that she would then go to school, to now - she doesn't want to get up.

Similarly, Parent 7LL1, whose child had suspected attention difficulties, stated: "And I can tell he doesn't like it [online learning] because [child 3] always asks me 'When are we going to school? When are we going to school?'"

Parent 8LL0, whose relationship with her children's teacher had worsened during the pandemic due to communication issues, had concerns about the virtual classroom environment. She described her child's reaction to not being able to express herself in French, perhaps due to having less one-on-one instruction:

> When my daughter asks a question, she's scared to ask because she doesn't want to get yelled at. So, we would ask, and they [the teacher] would say, 'ask in French.' But she doesn't know how to ask in French … or maybe she does, I don't know. She would just be like, 'Forget it. I don't want to ask anymore.' You could tell something's wrong, and you could tell she wants to ask, but she just feels discouraged. (Parent 8LL0)

A number of parents felt their "teaching" role changed the nature of their interactions with their children. Parent 6LL1 said she frequently "nagged" her daughter to complete her work. In addition, her daughter, who already had suspected socio-emotional issues, regressed emotionally during online schooling, needing to sleep with her mother more often and craving attention.

Adapting to Online Learning

Although Parent 4LM2 reported that her children preferred learning from home, most parents found online learning difficult, particularly when transitioning from an in-person to a virtual classroom environment. Difficulties were reflected in children often not being fully engaged in the learning process, being bored with the format and the material being poorly organized. This quote discusses these concerns as experienced by a child with suspected social–emotional difficulties:

> Because she's not engaged in virtual learning. I know she's not because I have to listen to her every day. Half the time I'm walking through, we have a very small space, and she's doing something completely different. The work is never finished. I'm constantly nagging her. So, what are you grading her on? I honestly have no idea how she's doing right now. I'm terrified for next year. (Parent 6LL1)

This quote from Parent 6LL1 also exemplifies the feelings of some parents that the transition process itself was disorganized, with little clear direction provided to parents and students about what they needed to learn or how they could demonstrate mastery. As a result, children would often not complete the assigned work. Similarly, Parent 7LL1 described how distracted her child with attentional difficulties was: "Because when he is at home, you see there are a lot of toys around him at home here, so he wants to do whatever he wants to do. … You know, it's very hard". Overall, children had difficulty adjusting to online learning due to a lack of engagement, difficulty sustaining attention and poor organization.

Parents' Experiences

Participants also spoke at length about how their children's transition to online learning impacted them. They discussed the impact on their own work schedules, their dual role as both a parent and a teacher, and the costs involved with access to technology and obtaining French resources. However, the most prominent theme was juggling their parental duties while taking on many educational support duties for their children. The most discussed topics in this subtheme included the educational strategies parents used and the teaching dynamics, their French language abilities and their communication with their children's teachers.

Impact on Parents' Work

Parents frequently talked about the impact of asynchronous learning on parents' work. One parent quit her job to support her children's learning at home, a privilege many parents cannot afford: "The pandemic has affected us all in different ways, and I left my job in the spring, but what that allowed for was so much more dedicated time to focus with them" (Parent 1MH1). Parents who worked from home said they were often interrupted by requests to explain assignments or help children with their lessons. Indeed, some children came to see their parents as the go-to person for their schoolwork:

> She's left alone a lot to just sort of figure it out. She came to me and interrupted a work call to tell me it was my responsibility to teach her subtraction. Or maybe it was division, … division in French, and I was like, no, not my responsibility. It's the middle of the day, you need to go back to your teacher and ask her to explain to you what it is that she's wanting from you. (Parent 6LL1)

On the other hand, parents who continued to work outside the home expressed guilt that they were not able to be home to help their children during class time:

> It's mostly because I can't be there to support her when I'm working. It makes me feel really guilty. My mom watches her, but my mom doesn't even know how to use a computer. She doesn't know French either, so that's difficult. (Parent 8LL0)

These three quotes demonstrate how SES impacted the online experiences of parents and children. Parent 1MH1 was able to quit her job during the pandemic because her husband worked full-time and was able to support them financially. Parents 6LL1 and 8LL0 were single parents and did not have this luxury, which impacted their ability to work with their children and support them when they struggled academically. SEN also seemed to impact parents' work situations. Of the five families who had at least one child with SEN, two chose to pause (4LM2) or quit their jobs to stay home with their children to provide educational and emotional support (1MH1). These mothers had a partner who worked through the pandemic.

Parent as Teacher

Strategies and Dynamics

Parental assistance with online schooling was not a formal expectation or requirement by the teachers or the schools. However, in reality, parents took on an educator role, monitoring their children's progress and supporting them when they struggled. Parents developed a variety of strategies to do this, such as developing homework schedules, asking children to read and write in French every day, and securing educational materials such as French reading programmes or French books from the library for their children to use. Parent 3HH0, who had typically developing children in FI explained:

> I realized how much he was struggling with this reading. I found this online program and we did it every single day and worked away at that. It was kind of like going back to the basics and helping him figure out how to sound out words.

Consistent with previous research (Garbe et al., 2020), many parents felt that more homework and the use of textbooks would have helped parents to monitor their children's progress and support their learning more effectively. According to Parent 2MH1: "The biggest challenge is that you don't see the progress and you can't evaluate the work. … And I honestly believe that textbooks and worksheets are the answer". Similarly, Parent 5MM0 felt that a French textbook that outlined the learning objectives and presented the material would have helped her work more effectively with her children and better understand intended learning outcomes.

Parents' French Language Abilities

Past research has shown that FI parents are concerned that their French knowledge limits their ability to support their children's learning at the best of times (Selvachandran et al., 2022). This concern was exacerbated during the pandemic as children's schooling went online: "I would need to explain [to] him what this is about, like the math background, … and then translate it to French. But since I'm not speaking [*sic*] French, … from March to September, we just lost everything" (Parent 5MM0).

Even when French resources were provided, they were intended for Francophone children and, therefore, were difficult to use. Parent 8LL0 expressed this frustration with the quality of the resources provided:

> I know, there's a lot of access to French resources. It's just sometimes I get stuck and I'm like, how do you do this? How do you play this game? She asks me for help, and I don't know how to help her because it's in French. (Parent 8LL0)

Many parents used Google Translate to help them overcome their French language challenges. Parent 6LL1 referred to this as "double duty" – translating first, then helping her child with homework, something that most parents of children in the English stream did not need to do. Parent 2MH1 told her son to use Google Translate himself rather than asking her for help because his French skills were better than hers. Overall, parents' lack of French proficiency was considered a major barrier to helping children succeed during online learning and made a difficult task even more challenging.

Communication with Teachers

The interviewed parents discussed the performance of teachers during the pandemic. In particular, teachers' ability to communicate effectively with parents and students and their use of teaching strategies were described.

> Her teacher was amazing, her grade one teacher. She would just communicate, and she would talk to me about her strengths … and weaknesses and what we should work on. She suggested, just keep reading to her, make sure she reads French every day, even though she doesn't understand it. (Parent 8LL0)

While all parents had the contact information of their children's teachers, they were not always able to establish reliable and beneficial communication. Most parents stated that teachers rarely communicated with them about their children's performance, which was particularly concerning for parents who had children with known or suspected SEN. We did not specifically query whether this was a significant deviation compared to communication before online learning, but parents certainly mentioned that communication was more challenging during online learning. Due to the lack of communication about their child's progress, parents felt unable to assess their children's progress themselves, given the fact that they did not speak French fluently. Consequently, most parents were unsure how their children were doing in the programme.

Cost

Access and Technology

In order to participate in online learning, children needed access to computers or iPads. The parents from high or mid-SES households did not report difficulties accessing these devices, and in some cases, they obtained more devices than they needed. For example, Parent 1MH1 purchased an Android tablet for each of her children and still received two iPads from the TDSB. However, lower-income families relied more on TDSB-sourced technology. When the laptops broke or malfunctioned, certain families were left in a difficult situation (Parent 7LL1). Some parents were able to purchase new laptops for their children in these situations, while others could not.

Internet access also proved to be an issue for many, especially when multiple people were online simultaneously. One parent (4LM2) described her inability to access instructional French YouTube videos provided to FI parents because of country-specific access restrictions. Although the parent did not elaborate as to why this occurred, it is possible that teachers and schools felt rushed to provide French resources to families during this time, resulting in inaccessible websites.

Parent-Sourced French Resources

Parents 5MM0 and 8LL0 felt that the loss of the school library with its free access to French books negatively impacted their children's ability to acquire French reading skills. Parents felt that the resources they obtained from their children's teachers and schools were not sufficient to support French language learning and sought to supplement their child's learning with additional French resources appropriate to their child's age or developmental level.

The type of resources parents sourced differed depending on the family's unique financial situation. Some obtained French workbooks or watched French-language programmes through the Canadian Broadcasting Company or Television Ontario. Other parents from financially secure households hired French tutors:

> We actually started getting him a virtual tutor. We know somebody in Europe ... and she has virtual classes with both of them one hour a week, every week, and they do some work. I don't think that's enough, to be honest with you, but at least it's something that we are kind of starting with. (Parent 2MH1)

Discussion

This study explored the impact of online learning during the COVID-19 pandemic, as experienced by eight families whose children were enrolled in a Canadian FI programme in the TDSB. All interviewees were mothers who played a primary role in supporting their children's online learning. The interviewed mothers discussed the strengths and challenges of online learning for themselves and their children.

The most commonly cited benefit of online learning was children's improvement in technology skills, including navigating computers and tablets and learning how to use web-based applications such as Google Classroom. Technology skills are increasingly important in both higher education and in the workforce, and a head start in acquiring tech literacy is arguably the most significant benefit of virtual schooling. For parents with children with special needs (e.g. 1MH1 and 4LM2), the additional one-on-one time spent with their children also proved beneficial, especially for parents who had the opportunity to quit their jobs and stay home. Another cited benefit of online learning was the increase in web-based educational resources to help students keep up with French reading, purchased by the school.

Despite the mentioned benefits, the interviewed mothers in the current study discussed numerous challenges of online learning. Experiences were in some ways similar to those reported for English classrooms, such as the negative impact on children's physical and mental health and parents' difficulty in juggling work and their children's schoolwork while working from home (Garbe et al., 2020). In addition, parents often felt a lack of communication from the teachers and the school regarding their children's progress and curriculum expectations. However, we found that the unique nature of the FI programme posed additional challenges compared to regular English stream programmes.

For example, parents highlighted the lack of French language input in a virtual classroom as a major problem, which could partially explain previous findings showing reduced French language vocabulary development compared to pre-pandemic levels (Abuosbeh et al., 2024).

It is important to note that the online format was much more challenging for teacher–student interactions compared to in-person schooling, particularly in the FI programme. Although French language instruction challenges existed prior to the pandemic, our interviews demonstrated that online learning was an additional barrier for students to develop their verbal French skills due to limited individualized time with the teacher and fewer French conversations with peers. As one parent noted, teachers would often resort to speaking in English when students struggled to understand instructions. It is important to consider that students in the English stream had the benefit of sustained literacy education and language development in the form of conversations with families and television programmes and other media. The parents' lack of French knowledge, combined with limited access to French media in Ontario, makes maintaining the language challenging outside of the classroom setting.

We queried whether experiences differed for diverse students in the programme. In many ways, interviewees from diverse families discussed similar issues, such as delays in their children's French progress and difficulties in supporting their children's French homework. While all parents struggled to ensure their children were supported, there was evidence that parents of children with SEN experience particular pressures in this regard. For example, two mothers paused or quit their jobs to better support their children with SEN. Parents reported that they and their children suffered worse physical and mental health throughout this period, which was exacerbated by the challenge of parents balancing the role of teacher and parent. As shown in previous studies (Asbury et al., 2021; Neece et al., 2020), the pandemic exaggerated the difficulty of accessing internal and external resources for students with SEN. Families of children with SEN often feel that they must secure external resources, such as tutors, assessments and diagnoses, even before the pandemic, due to a dearth of SEN support in FI (Mady & Muhling, 2017; Selvachandran et al., 2022).

Regarding SES, not surprisingly, access to resources was an area where low-income families were adversely affected. While school boards provided devices and internet to families who needed them, these devices sometimes broke or malfunctioned and were not replaced in a timely fashion. Low-income families, therefore, struggled to acquire and maintain functional devices critical for online learning. Given that access to technology and the internet facilitate learning and increase student engagement (Domina et al., 2021), a lack of reliable devices or internet access creates inequalities in the quality of education, which can exacerbate existing disparities in student performance.

Some families (e.g. 5MM0 and 8LL0) also had difficulty in accessing resources such as tutors, French books and supplies beyond those provided by the school. As previously mentioned, many parents felt the school board provided helpful online educational resources to support French learning during this period, such as Raz Kids, Boukili and Lalilo. While helpful, access to these websites does not mean it was enough, however, to sustain French education during this period. Additionally, although these online resources were provided during the pandemic, according to our participants, they have since been withdrawn by the schools when students returned to in-person learning.

Unfortunately, the lack of access to free resources is an ongoing issue for low-SES families in the FI programme. As previously mentioned, the FI programme has a reputation for elitism as it allows families with the financial means to keep their children in the programme through additional help such as tutors and extra-curricular activities, disadvantaging low-income students and students of colour (Kunnas, 2019). Low-income families often feel that they have no other choice other than to withdraw their children who are struggling from the programme. In the present study, we found differences between low SES families who struggled during this period due to financial constraints (e.g. 6LL1 and 8LL0) and higher SES families who were able to provide additional support for their children during this time (e.g. 1MH1 and 4LM2).

All of these highlighted challenges (i.e. limited access to French resources, difficulty sustaining French input and output, parents' difficulty in supporting their children's French language education, increased difficulties for low SES families and students with SEN) reflect issues within the educational system that existed in a pre-pandemic world. While online learning highlighted and worsened some of these challenges, many of these difficulties were voiced by parents regarding FI education even before the pandemic (Cepin, 2012; Wise, 2011). Therefore, it is critical that these concerns are addressed in the future through policy changes, both in the case of another global emergency and to improve the success and equity of the FI programme for future students.

Policy Implications and Recommendations

On May 5th, 2023, the World Health Organization officially announced the end of the COVID-19 global health emergency. Although students are now back in school, the long-term health effects of COVID-19 are uncertain, and other pandemics may occur. Since it is possible that other pandemics or emergency stay-at-home orders may occur in the future, it is vital to be prepared and learn from past experiences with virtual schooling. For students who obtain their academic instruction in their non-dominant language, such as those in the FI programme, school boards and teachers must be prepared to provide additional support to these students (e.g. clear and consistent communication from the school and teacher, a variety of multi-modal resources that can be accessed from home for free, in-school interventions that are created specifically for FI students). The participants' concerns that online FI learning experiences negatively impacted their children's French language learning echoed reports from Canada and the United States of curriculum delays during the pandemic in other subject areas (Kuhfeld et al., 2020). It is unclear whether such delays in learning the required curriculum will be overcome with the return to in-person programming.

In the future, online learning in FI would benefit from an emphasis on second language exposure through reading and listening. This could be fostered through enhanced student–teacher interactions and greater access to French resources, such as workbooks or additional help in the form of school-funded tutoring. It would be beneficial for school boards to prepare FI curriculum materials that are suitable for online learning in advance, including access to educational programmes. These preparations would set the groundwork for successful online learning and teaching in the future, either in the event of another global emergency or if virtual schooling becomes more commonplace and accessible, such as for students with disabilities.

Furthermore, it is particularly important to provide extra support for students with SEN. For example, access to timely assessments, interventions in the form of extra individualized support, and accommodations should continue to be provided to students in the FI programme without interruption. For low SES families and communities in FI, resource inequities still exist despite current policies that are intended to narrow the gap (Learning Opportunities Index, 2020). In our interviews, some parents discussed obtaining access to online educational resources that helped, such as Raz Kids. Continued access to these materials, even in the post-COVID era, is vital in ensuring that students from low SES backgrounds can continue to succeed in the FI programme.

Limitations and Future Directions

Several limitations should be acknowledged in this study. This study investigated the perspectives of parents; future studies should expand our understanding of the pandemic's effects on the FI programme by seeking the perspectives of teachers and administrators. It is important to note that teachers and administrators had their own immense challenges during the transition to online learning, including navigating the technological aspects of the transition, creating virtual lesson plans, managing student behaviour and engagement, and balancing their responsibilities with their own families.

In addition, the number of participants from various diverse backgrounds was limited. Unfortunately, developmental research often suffers from a self-selection effect in sampling; parents with more motivation and time may be more willing to participate in a research study and undergo a lengthy interview process. A larger sample size could expand our understanding of how virtual learning in the context of FI affects students from racialized backgrounds and immigrant families, especially those who do not speak English or French at home.

It is important to note that three out of the eight families interviewed came from homes where neither English nor French was spoken as a native language. We did not see a substantial difference in the reported experience of students who spoke a different language at home relative to others in this study, although we largely attribute this to the fact that all the parents needed to speak English to participate. Still, it is possible that these families were not impacted more than English-speaking families, consistent with previous research (Bild & Swain, 1989).

Importantly, we did not ask the parents directly whether they felt that certain factors (such as being in a lower SES or having a child with an SEN) affected their experience. Instead, our questions revolved around the shift to online learning for FI students during the pandemic. Through our conversations with the parents, the impacts of SES and SEN on these families' and children's experiences were made apparent. However, future studies should explicitly ask participants how SES and SEN play a role in their experience and their children's success in the programme.

Conclusion

In 2020, lockdown measures and school closures required students worldwide to move to virtual schooling. Although such measures helped keep families safe during the pandemic, online learning posed many challenges to all students. However, some students were disproportionately affected.

The current study interviewed parents in Ontario, Canada, whose children are enrolled in the FI programme in the TDSB. Consistent with previous research on the effect of the COVID-19 pandemic on children's education, the parents in the current study voiced many of the same benefits (e.g. improvement in technology skills, additional school resources, focused attention) and challenges (e.g. impact on children's well-being, adapting to online learning, impact on parents' work, having to take an active role in their child's education) as parents with children in regular English programming. However, for FI students, the language of instruction at school is not their dominant language, making it more difficult to maintain sufficient French input and output outside of a traditional classroom setting.

In their attempts to secure French resources and obtain extra support, families from low SES backgrounds or with children with SEN faced additional challenges. Parents expressed that the free resources provided by the schools were not sufficient to sustain French literacy during this period. Low SES households struggled to juggle work demands and their children's educations, while some parents in high SES households quit their jobs to dedicate their time to helping their children succeed, in addition to securing French tutors and additional external resources. Students with SEN, particularly those with mental health challenges such as anxiety, fared worse in an online learning environment.

As we move towards an increasingly digital age, there is a need to understand how educational systems can change and adapt. We hope that highlighting the benefits and challenges communicated by parents will help to guide future decisions regarding online learning, particularly in FI programmes. Future policy should focus on eliminating the additional barriers encountered by children who come from low-income families or who have SEN.

References

Abuosbeh, Z., Burchell, D., Krenca, K., & Chen, X. (2024). The impact of online learning during the pandemic on language and reading performance in English–French bilingual children. *Journal of Research in Reading*, *47*(3), 1–18. https://doi.org/10.1111/1467-9817.12450.

Asbury, K., Fox, L., Deniz, E., Code, A., & Toseeb, U. (2021). How is COVID-19 affecting the mental health of children with special educational needs and disabilities and their families? *Journal of Autism and Developmental Disorders*, *51*(5), 1772–1780. https://doi.org/10.1007/s10803-020-04577-2.

Bild, E. R., & Swain, M. (1989). Minority language students in a French immersion programme: Their French proficiency. *Journal of Multilingual & Multicultural Development*, *10*(3), 255–274. https://doi.org/10.1080/01434632.1989.9994377.

Braun, V., & Clarke, V. (2006). Using thematic analysis in psychology. *Qualitative Research in Psychology*, *3*(2), 77–101.

Cepin, J. J. (2012). *Spaces of Option and Opportunity in Education: Equity Issues and French Immersion Programming in Toronto*. Thesis, York University.

Domina, T., Renzulli, L., Murray, B., Garza, A. N., & Perez, L. (2021). Remote or removed: Predicting successful engagement with online learning during COVID-19. *Socius*, *7*, 1–15. https://doi.org/10.1177/2378023120988200.

Dresing, T., Pehl, T., & Schmieder, C. (2015). *Manual (on) Transcription: Transcription Conventions, Software Guides and Practical Hints for Qualitative Researchers* (3rd English Ed). Marburg.

Egbo, B. (2009). *Teaching for Diversity in Canadian Schools*. Pearson Prentice Hall.

Fontenelle-Tereshchuk, D. (2021). 'Homeschooling' and the COVID-19 crisis: The insights of parents on curriculum and remote learning. *Interchange*, *52*(2), 167–191. https://doi.org/10.1007/s10780-021-09420-w.

Garbe, A., Ogurlu, U., Logan, N., & Cook, P. (2020). COVID-19 and remote learning: Experiences of parents with children during the pandemic. *American Journal of Qualitative Research*, *4*(3), 45–65. https://doi.org/10.29333/ajqr/8471.

Genesee, F., & Lindholm-Leary, K. (2021). The suitability of dual language education for diverse students: An overview of research in Canada and the United States. *Journal of Immersion and Content-Based Language Education*, *9*(2), 164–192. https://doi.org/10.1075/jicb.21001.gen.

Government of Ontario. (2022). *Public Health Measures and Advice.* Retrieved from https://www.ontario.ca/page/public-health-measures-and-advice.

Hipfner-Boucher, K., Burchell, D., & Chen, X. (2022). *L2 Reading Development in Minority Language Speaker* [Chapter Accepted]. Ontario Institute for Studies in Education, University of Toronto.

Kaffenberger, M. (2021). Modelling the long-run learning impact of the Covid-19 learning shock: Actions to (more than) mitigate loss. *International Journal of Educational Development, 81*, Article 102326. https://doi.org/10.1016/j.ijedudev.2020.102326.

Kay-Raining Bird, E., Genesee, F., Sutton, A., Chen, X., Oracheski, J., Pagan, S., Squires, B., Burchell, D., & Sorenson Duncan, T. (2021). Access and outcomes of children with special education needs in early French immersion. *Journal of Immersion and Content-Based Language Education, 9*(2), 193–222. https://doi.org/10.1075/jicb.20012.kay.

Kuhfeld, M., Soland, J., Tarasawa, B., Johnson, A., Ruzek, E., & Liu, J. (2020). Projecting the potential impact of COVID-19 school closures on academic achievement. *Educational Researcher, 49*(8), 549–565. https://doi.org/10.3102/0013189X20965918.

Kunnas, R. M. (2019). *Inequities in Black et Blanc: Textual Constructions of the French Immersion Student* [Unpublished Master's thesis]. University of Toronto.

Lazaruk, W. (2007). Linguistic, academic, and cognitive benefits of French immersion. *Canadian Modern Language Review, 63*(5), 605–627.

Lindholm-Leary, K., & Genesee, F. (2014). Student outcomes in one-way, two-way, and Indigenous language immersion education. *Journal of Immersion and Content-Based Language Education, 2*(2), 165–180. https://doi.org/10.1075/jicb.2.2.01lin.

MacDonald, M., & Hill, C. (2022). The educational impact of the Covid-19 rapid response on teachers, students, and families: Insights from British Columbia, Canada. *Prospects, 51*(4), 627–641. https://doi.org/10.1007/s11125-020-09527-5.

Mady, C., & Muhling, S. (2017). Instructional supports for students with special education needs in French as a second language education: A review of Canadian empirical literature. *Journal of Education and Learning, 6*(3), 14–22. https://doi.org/10.5539/jel.v6n3p14.

Neece, C., McIntyre, L. L., & Fenning, R. (2020). Examining the impact of COVID-19 in ethnically diverse families with young children with intellectual and developmental disabilities. *Journal of Intellectual Disability Research, 64*(10), 739–749. https://doi.org/10.1111/jir.12769.

Rehner, K., & Mougeon, R. (2003). The effect of educational input on the development of sociolinguistic competence by French immersion students: The case of expressions of consequence in spoken French. *The Journal of Educational Thought (JET)/Revue de la Pensée Educative*, 259–281.

Schleicher, A. (2020). *The Impact of COVID-19 on Education: Insights from "Education at a Glance 2020"*. OECD Publishing.

Selvachandran, J., Kay-Raining Bird, E., DeSousa, J., & Chen, X. (2022). Special education needs in French immersion: A parental perspective of supports and challenges. *International Journal of Bilingual Education and Bilingualism, 25*(3), 1120–1136. https://doi.org/10.1080/13670050.2020.1742650.

Sinay, E. (2010). Programs of choice in the TDSB: Characteristics of students in French immersion, alternative schools, and other specialized schools and programs. Toronto District School Board. https://books.scholarsportal.info/uri/ebooks/ebooks0/gibson_cppc/2014-09-25/1/10886170.

Teotonio, I. (2023, April 12). Parents threaten legal action for TDSB error that excluded racialized, disabled and LGBTQ students from alternative school lottery. *Toronto Star*. Retrieved 25 July 2024, from https://www.thestar.com/news/gta/parents-threaten-legal-action-for-tdsb-error-that-excluded-racialized-disabled-and-lgbtq-students-from/article_58e1dd98-f5ab-5985-9857-7dd93b5ac40e.html.

Toronto District School Board. (2020). *The 2020 Learning Opportunities Index: Questions and Answers*. TDSB Research Reports. Retrieved 18 December 2022, from https://www.tdsb.on.ca/Portals/research/docs/reports/LOI2020.pdf.

Wise, N. (2011). Access to special education for exceptional students in French immersion programs: An equity issue. *Canadian Journal of Applied Linguistics*, *14*(1), 177–193.

Yoon, E. S., Grima, V., DeWiele, C. E. B., & Skelton, L. (2022). The impact of school choice on school (re) segregation: Settler-colonialism, critical geography and Bourdieu. *Comparative Education*, *58*(1), 52–71.

· 2 ·

THE RIPPLE EFFECT: POST-SECONDARY STUDENTS, SYSTEMIC INEQUITY, AND THE COVID-19 PANDEMIC

Serenity Friskie and Sunny Manhas

While the COVID-19 virus does not discriminate, the COVID-19 pandemic has exposed the deep and pervasive systemic inequities that shape Canadian society and social relations. Across many sectors, the pandemic has also exacerbated pre-existing inequities among marginalized groups, particularly those with intersecting social identities. As a result, the pandemic has brought conversations of equity to the forefront of political and social discourse.

Post-secondary students were acutely impacted during the early stages of the pandemic, grappling with disrupted studies, sudden job losses, and evaporating career opportunities (The Daily, 2020). However, the burden of this crisis did not fall equally. Marginalized students – including racialized communities, students with disabilities, international students, and those from low-income backgrounds – were disproportionately affected. These students faced compounded barriers, such as inadequate access to digital resources, heightened financial precarity, unstable housing, and a lack of culturally relevant mental health support (Jones et al., 2021). The pandemic exposed and deepened pre-existing inequities, underscoring the urgent need to address these systemic injustices. Examining the COVID-19 pandemic's impact on marginalized students is crucial for understanding how post-secondary institutions can promote equity within their communities. The pandemic has exacerbated existing inequalities, particularly affecting students from racialized backgrounds, low-income families, and those with disabilities (Blanco et al., 2020; Canadian Alliance of Student Associations, 2021). Many of these students face intensified challenges, such as financial instability and mental health issues, which have been worsened by the shift to remote learning, revealing disparities in technology access and resulting in significant academic setbacks (Sweeney et al., 2021; Kraft & Simon, 2021). To effectively support these students, institutions must adopt inclusive policies that prioritize mental health resources and academic support while fostering a sense of community (Canadian Federation of Students, 2021). Engaging actively with marginalized voices will enable post-secondary institutions to develop strategies that address both the immediate challenges posed by the pandemic and the need for long-term equity and inclusion.

To explore the impacts of the COVID-19 pandemic on post-secondary students, we analyse five qualitative interviews conducted in the Lower Mainland of British Columbia as part of a pilot study examining the social impacts of the COVID-19 pandemic on students. We discuss pre-existing obstacles for post-secondary students, such as financial barriers and mental health challenges. We also investigate students' experiences of gender-based violence during the COVID-19 pandemic, which the World Health Organization referred to as "the shadow pandemic" (UN Women, 2020; UN Women, 2021). We direct attention to the experiences of post-secondary students with racialized identities and, more specifically, the experiences of Black and Indigenous post-secondary students.

In our analysis, we reflected on our own positionalities and maintained awareness of participants' social locations, which includes intersecting factors such as race, gender, socio-economic status, and geographic location. Keeping this in mind, we want to stress that the goal of this chapter is not to exploit the narratives of marginalized communities but to uplift and amplify their lived experiences. In this chapter, "marginalized peoples" refers to individuals and groups who experience systemic disadvantages based on various intersecting factors such as race, ethnicity, gender, socio-economic status, and sexual orientation. These communities often face barriers that limit their access to essential resources and opportunities, leading to social, economic, and political exclusion (Crenshaw, 1989; Christoffersen & Emejulu, 2023; hooks, 2000). By focusing on their lived experiences, the chapter aims to support and amplify the voices of these groups, advocating for social justice and equity. This approach seeks to shift narratives from exploitation to empowerment, emphasizing the importance of recognizing and validating the realities of marginalized communities (Mansbridge & Morris, 2001). Importantly, we found that the pandemic significantly contributed to complex challenges that hindered the success of post-secondary students, especially marginalized students. In the sections that follow, we investigate some of the many ways in which the COVID-19 pandemic had a ripple effect, exacerbating system oppressions that marginalized students experience during their post-secondary schooling.

Situating Ourselves

Before we begin, we would like to introduce ourselves and our relationship to this work. We are both post-secondary students, and the COVID-19 pandemic impacted us in unique ways. Our individual experiences do not disappear when conducting this research, and we feel it is important to recognize how our experiences informed our analysis and are reflected in participants' stories.

About the Author: Serenity Friskie

My name is Seren Friskie, and I am an Indigenous, queer-identifying woman and the only member of my immediate family who has attended post-secondary. I identify myself as a queer ethnic anomaly, with an ancestry mixed with Coast Salish, Cree, German, and French roots. I currently live on the unsurrendered, unceded, and occupied territories of the Sḵwx̱wú7mesh (Squamish), Stó:lō and Səl'ílwətaʔ/Selilwitulh (Tsleil-Waututh) and xʷməθkʷəy̓əm (Musqueam) Nations.

As a full-time student who is working three jobs and has obligations to provide financial and emotional support to my family, I have been affected by the COVID-19 pandemic in numerous ways. I lost two family members, including one to an overdose. Many of us are facing an affordable housing crisis, where unhoused people are being unethically targeted in tent camp raids (Takeuchi, 2020). We have people dying on our streets due to fentanyl-contaminated drug supplies that have pushed overdose deaths to levels never seen before in British Columbia (BC Centre for Disease Control, 2020). We have shed tears of fear, worry, and loss. The COVID-19 pandemic has been a time of tremendous struggle for us, and it makes me question who our government prioritizes and who they believe deserves support. We have heard slogans like "we are all in this together" and seen local expressions of solidarity (Watson, 2020), but who actually receives support, resources, and attention in Canada? This is where my research interests lie.

As explained above, the pandemic has exposed and exacerbated violence, oppression, and inequities in Canadian society. I felt compelled to conduct this research due to my own post-secondary institution's lack of response and support, and the hurdles I was facing. This research presented me with the opportunity to connect with peers from marginalized communities, elevate their voices, and shed light on their lived experiences. Despite the challenges, this research has inspired me to continue to push for changes in social policy and advocate for marginalized people.

About the Author: Sunny Manhas

My name is Sunny Manhas, and I am a queer person of colour who has spent the last several years working with marginalized communities. In the mid 1970s, my family immigrated from Punjab, India to what is colonially known as Canada. I am a settler on the traditional, ancestral, and stolen lands of the Sḵwx̱wú7mesh (Squamish), Stó:lō and Səl̓ílwətaʔ/Selilwitulh (Tsleil-Waututh) and xʷməθkʷəy̓əm (Musqueam) Nations, which are now referred to as Vancouver. At the time of writing this chapter, I am completing a Bachelor of Social Work at the University of British Columbia, working at two organizations that each focus on addressing gender-based violence, and volunteering with a grassroots community organization that responds to the housing crisis and the opioid epidemic.

There are several reasons why I was interested in researching the experiences of post-secondary marginalized students during the COVID-19 pandemic. First, I witnessed my peers enduring challenging circumstances. Second, I was struggling. Third, I have a deep regard for scholarly and professional approaches rooted in intersectionality and anti-oppressive practices, and this research was an opportunity to prioritize the experiences of systemically oppressed students in the pandemic. My goal for this research is for our findings to inform institutional responses and improve the circumstances, supports, and systems that are meant to serve students experiencing oppression in the post-secondary environment.

Method

This chapter examines five in-depth qualitative interviews conducted in August 2020 with marginalized post-secondary students living in the Lower Mainland of British Columbia. All participants were enrolled full-time or part-time in university classes during the 2019–2020 academic year. The research was approved by the Douglas College Research Ethics Board and all participants signed an informed consent form. Interviews lasted about 45–60 minutes and were held via Zoom. We recorded the video and audio of the interviews and transcribed them using both transcription software and traditional transcription methods. Due to the sensitive nature of the topics discussed in some of the interviews, we presented participants with options for support through local and provincial resources. All participants received a $10 gift card as compensation.

Participants were recruited for one month by word of mouth and referrals from faculty members, peer students and student advisers. This non-representative, convenience sampling method was determined to be the most appropriate recruitment approach since the objective of the study was to generate an in-depth understanding of lived experience (Lavrakas, 2008). To this end, the findings presented in this chapter are not reflective of the experience of all marginalized post-secondary students in the Lower Mainland of British Columbia, or in Canada more generally. Instead, the findings provide insight into the unique experiences of these participants as they confront and navigate barriers, stigma, discrimination, and other challenges in post-secondary educational institutions and society. The interviews provided a cathartic opportunity for participants to reflect on and share their lived experiences, and they offer a snapshot into the lives of marginalized post-secondary students.

The interviews explored participants' experiences as students both before and during the COVID-19 pandemic. Participants discussed the complexities of post-secondary student life, talking about a variety of topics including their sense of self and identity, socio-economic situation, accessibility needs, and mental health. We also asked them to describe their experiences during the COVID-19 pandemic, as our questions focused on participants' social locations and the challenges they experienced during that time. During the interviews, participants were asked to self-identify and, as such, we list participants' identities as they were presented to us.

The five participant interviews we examine in this chapter are: (1) Mei, a queer, 24 year old, middle class, Chinese, cisgender woman living in Vancouver who was a full-time, fourth year undergraduate student doing a degree in gender, sexuality, and women's studies; (2) Garrett, a heterosexual, 51 year old, working class, Indigenous man living in Vancouver who was a full-time, second year undergraduate student studying psychology; (3) Parminder, a heterosexual, 20 year old, middle class, Indian man living in Surrey who was a full-time, second year undergraduate student studying psychology; (4) Dion, a heterosexual, 21 year old, middle class, Nigerian woman living in Vancouver who was a part-time, third year undergraduate student studying business; and (5) Kelsie, a heterosexual, 34 year old, middle class, white, cisgender woman with a disability, living in Coquitlam who was a full-time, second year student studying psychology. All names have been changed to protect the identity of the participants.

We analysed the interview data through the lenses of decolonial thought (Torres, 2017), intersectionality (Crenshaw, 1989, 1990, 2017), and anti-oppressive practices (Burke & Harrison, 1998) to explore the ways in which students experienced barriers before and during the COVID-19 pandemic. Integrating decolonial thought, intersectionality, and anti-oppressive practices into the analysis of interview data creates a robust framework for understanding the complexities of participants' experiences, particularly those from marginalized communities. In analysing interview data through the lenses of decolonial thought, intersectionality, and anti-oppressive practices, we gain a comprehensive understanding of the complexities faced by marginalized communities. Decolonial thought critiques the enduring impacts of colonialism on knowledge production and emphasizes the importance of Indigenous epistemologies (Torres, 2017). Intersectionality, introduced by Crenshaw (1989), explores how overlapping identities shape distinct experiences of privilege and oppression, revealing the multifaceted nature of systemic inequalities. Furthermore, anti-oppressive practices focus on dismantling power imbalances and advocating for the inclusion of marginalized voices in decision-making processes, ultimately promoting social justice (Dominelli, 2002; Mackenzie & Fagan, 2018). Together, these frameworks illuminate the intricate dynamics of identity and oppression, guiding researchers toward more equitable and inclusive outcomes in their work.

We applied these theoretical frameworks to carefully consider salient points from participants' experience and recognize repetitions across the interviews. As such, we conducted in-depth readings of the transcripts and identified common themes across participants' experiences, as well as specific examples related to each participant's unique and intersectional social location. We contextualized our findings within systems that afford some people power and marginalize others, such as whiteness and systemic racism, misogyny, heteronormativity, colonization, and xenophobia, among others. In our analysis below, we provide participant quotes to highlight their experiences and expose systems of inequity and institutional barriers.

Barriers Experienced by Post-Secondary Students During COVID-19

Although trials and tribulations are not new to students – many of whom intend to establish a life path or a transition to a new career – numerous barriers have been exacerbated by the COVID-19 pandemic. In this section, we discuss some of these barriers, including mental health challenges, tuition and employment difficulties, and systemic inequities. All these barriers can affect students' academic success, personal relationships, and social connections as well as their prospects for employment after graduation.

Mental Health

Although students' mental health is critical to their well-being as well as their success in post-secondary education, it is common for post-secondary students to struggle with mental health challenges. Post-secondary students experience anxiety about academic performance, debt accumulation, tuition fees, and uncertainty about their future in the labour market after graduation (Kaniasty et al., 2014). Other research has shown that anxiety and depression are the two biggest concerns among students (Reetz et al., 2014).

Unfortunately, data indicate that such feelings have been on the rise. The Canadian Institute for Health Information found that emergency department mental health visits for patients aged 12–24 increased by 85 % from 2007 to 2012 (Mental Health Commission of Canada, 2012). By 2021, suicide accounted for 20% of deaths among youth aged 10–14, 28% among youth aged 15–19, and 24% among young adults aged 20–24 (Statistics Canada, 2026). More recently, in the early months of the COVID-19 pandemic in Canada, 27% of youth aged 15–24 reported symptoms of moderate to severe anxiety (Statistics Canada, 2020b). Emerging research continues to show that the pandemic has contributed to increased feelings of loneliness, stress, anxiety, and depression among university students, with a 2023 survey revealing that over 40% of students reported experiencing moderate to severe mental health concerns (Michigan Medicine, 2023). Participants in our study talked about feeling anxiety related to the pandemic. For example, Mei said:

> I'm super anxious about COVID. Even if I didn't feel like it was affecting anything, it obviously did. Like, the energy of the world right now is just so negative. It also made it a lot easier to just say "Oh I'm feeling anxious, can I get an extension?" That's really bad and I'm not saying that's what I did, but it was a true thing. My mom was really scared of having COVID-19 and was at home for a whole month. So there was just a lot of mental and emotional stress there already. So I'm not trying to take advantage of this, but I'm not *not* trying to take advantage of this. But I'm also stressed caring for my mom.

Mei was experiencing anxiety – first, related to the academic pressures of post-secondary education and second, related to concerns about family members' health and her caretaker responsibilities – both of which were exacerbated by the pandemic. In fact, Mei explained that these unrelenting stressors seriously impacted her ability to fully engage in life and school: "My anxiety kind of disables me sometimes."

Recent data suggests that the challenges Mei experienced were common among other post-secondary students during this time. Between 19 April 2020, and 1 May 2020, Statistics Canada collected data from over 100,000 post-secondary students and found that almost two-thirds of respondents were "very" or "extremely" concerned about the impact of the pandemic on their grades, while nearly half were worried about their inability to return to school in the next term (Statistics Canada, 2020a). Respondents also expressed being "very" or "extremely" concerned about using up their savings (68%), lacking job prospects (67%), and taking on more student debt (54%) as a result of the pandemic (Statistics Canada, 2020b). Another theme reflected in the data was the effect of social isolation on participants' mental health. Multiple participants described feeling frustrated and alone during the lockdown period in the early months of the pandemic – and they were not alone in feeling this way. While feelings of isolation are common for post-secondary students across Canada (Tang et al., 2019), the rapid spread of COVID-19 and the implementation of restrictions such as self-quarantine and social isolation contributed to a growing trend of loneliness (Banerjee & Rai, 2020). In fact, one study found that 54% of Canadians surveyed said that physical distancing left them feeling lonely or isolated (Bricker, 2020). All five of our participants stated that they endured a balancing act of adhering to public health recommendations while trying to maintain positive mental health. Kelsie said:

> We need to interact with one another. And it's like a way that we cope with all kinds of stress and not being able to do that very natural thing it just sucks. It just sucks. And it means that people, including myself, I'm making choices to put myself at a higher risk of contracting COVID-19 in order to, like, support my mental health.

Similarly, Parminder talked about feeling "cabin fever" because of social isolation. He also said that isolation impacted his ability to perform academically: "I enjoy having that [in-person social] interaction with people and I thrive on that to have my success. So, it becomes harder."

The pandemic was extremely isolating for participants and made them feel like they needed to choose between taking care of their mental health and protecting themselves – and others – from COVID-19. As such, our analysis exposes two other problems that post-secondary students endured during this time: the need to prioritize one type of health over another and, consequently, the implications of making such a decision. If they prioritized their mental health, this could be to the detriment to their physical health and the public's health. If they prioritized their physical health, it could be detrimental to their mental health. Such decisions were challenging for the post-secondary students in our study to make as they had to determine which aspects of their health (and other people's health) were most important.

Participants' mental health was also impacted by other factors. Mei said that, in addition to concerns about the COVID-19 virus, she was anxious about her work and her ability to pay tuition. Parminder echoed this sentiment and stated, "There's just a whole bunch of factors that we need to take in such as money, jobs, social interactions that can cause stress." Dion said that being a person of colour was an additional stressor which "leaked into" and affected her mental state. Although universities offer students mental health services, Dion explained that she had a hard time seeking out services during the pandemic:

> I'm just so exhausted, you know? I tried doing all the research. Like, I'm *so* exhausted by the end of the day from work and school. There should be a platform where they reach out to students and young adults, like Instagram or Facebook, where they just throw resources at you. I feel like that's a really good idea.

Like Dion, Mei talked about the exhaustion of working and attending school and said that she lacked the energy to reach out for support from professors or counselling services at her university. Mei recommended post-secondary institutions take a proactive rather than reactive approach to mental health services, so that the care comes to students.

The question then becomes: how can institutions offer comprehensive wellness and health services before a crisis occurs? Dion suggested using social media platforms to reach out to students: "I'll say Instagram was a resource. That was one of the things that kept me tuned in." Accounts like @FoundryBC (Foundry, n.d.) and @themindgeek (Crosby, n.d.) are two examples of resources that participants said offered students a variety of mental health supports, such as self-care tips, coping advice, and insight into issues like anxiety, depression, and stress. For Dion, social media provided mental health support during the pandemic – support that was more easily accessible than her institution's.

In recent years, Instagram has been utilized to raise awareness about mental health and illnesses, share treatment experiences, disseminate anti-stigma information, and provide anecdotal accounts (Gupta & Ariefdjohan, 2021). Dion was not alone; many Canadians turned to their devices to cope during the lockdown, resulting in a 10.5 % increase in social media use in July 2020 compared to July 2019 (Kemp, 2020). This suggests that many people turned to sites like Facebook or Instagram for various reasons, such as COVID-19 updates, entertainment, and socialization. The accessibility of social media platforms is important to keep in mind when considering how health services can be improved in the future, especially since students who sought counselling from post-secondary institutions experienced long wait times (British Columbia, 2020).

The Cost of Education

Post-secondary education is costly, and many students struggle to pay for tuition, housing, food, and other expenses. Before the pandemic, Garrett had trouble finding affordable housing when he relocated to British Columbia for school: "There are usually years on the waitlist [for social housing]. I'm single and I don't have any children so it's like, I'm at the bottom of the list." Kelsie said that, before COVID, she had to get a second job to pay for a diagnosis for her disability, which was required for academic accommodations at her institution. With the pandemic, students' financial situations have become more precarious. Dion noted that "international fees are super expensive" for non-Canadian students and that, since COVID hit, she needed to be more "astute with savings". Dion was already concerned about the financial costs related to being an international student, and her stress was exacerbated by the pandemic.

Students' financial circumstances can create barriers to their education, and these barriers have been exacerbated by the COVID-19 pandemic. They are not alone. Data from Statistics Canada (2020c) indicate that 51 % of students were "very" or "extremely" concerned about their ability to keep up with other bills and payments during the pandemic (Statistics Canada, 2020a). Mei, who was not working during the spring 2020 lockdown and lacked alternative options for income or economic support, explained that she began "sugaring" – a term she used to refer to being compensated for having sex – because she had to pay her tuition fees: "I need money to pay this because I don't have enough saved by now… I'm almost there but like I still only have two weeks left. And I am not able to make this amount." Mei's situation is not uncommon, as many post-secondary students engage in sex work because of financial concerns (Sanders & Hardy, 2015) and limited financial support (Sinacore et al., 2014). While more research is needed to understand how post-secondary students managed their financial responsibilities during the COVID-19 pandemic, Mei's experience reminds us of the accessibility and profitability of sex work during financially precarious times.

Sexual Violence

It is important to recognize that systemic inequities can exacerbate violence and harm against marginalized people – effects worsened by the COVID-19 pandemic. In Mei's case, one of her clients acted out against her by refusing to pay and sexually harassing her online. She explained, "I wouldn't call that violence necessarily, but I felt *assaulted* in a way." Mei felt unsafe, upset, and anxious as a result, feelings that were made worse by her history of sexual trauma and the effects of pandemic:

> I had a lot of anxiety, it just traumatized me. Because I have a lot of like, really shitty sexual assault background. So it just brought up things and my anxiety just spiked really high. And it was all during COVID and I couldn't go out. And it was all really bad because I wasn't thinking like, what if this guy has COVID.

Mei's experience exemplifies the "shadow pandemic", a term coined by the World Health Organization to highlight the surge in gender-based violence amid the COVID-19 crisis (UN Women, 2020). Prior to the pandemic, statistics indicated that approximately 30% of women aged 15 or older reported experiencing sexual assault at least once (Canadian Women's Foundation, 2021). The pandemic exacerbated these issues, with reports indicating that rates of domestic violence increased by 20 to 30% in various regions of Canada (Patel, 2020).

This rise in violence is not an isolated issue; it has been linked to various pandemic-related stressors, including economic uncertainty, social isolation, and increased time spent in the home with abusers (UN Women, 2021; Peterman et al., 2020). Reports from UN Women (2021) further emphasize that the pandemic has led to increased vulnerability for women and girls, particularly those in marginalized communities.

Research also suggests that support services for victims have been strained or inaccessible during the pandemic, making it more challenging for those experiencing violence to seek help (World Health Organization, 2021). This "shadow pandemic" underscores the urgent need for comprehensive policies and support systems to address and mitigate the impacts of gender-based violence, especially in the context of ongoing crises.

Although Mei is not alone in her experience, it is important to understand the structural factors that shaped her experience. Mei is a racialized queer woman who, like many other marginalized women, is a target of sexual violence because of their intersectional identities (Crenshaw, 1989). Racialized women and queer women experience elevated rates of sexual violence compared to white women and heterosexual women (Brennan, 2011; Scrim, 2017; Cotter, 2018; Logie et al., 2017). It is within this context that Mei experienced a violation of consent, which had considerable effects on her health, as she stated that she "felt traumatized and had multiple mental breakdowns". Mei, who had engaged in sex work to alleviate financial problems brought on by the pandemic, risked catching COVID-19 by engaging in sex work and experienced sexual harassment that caused her emotional distress – and was also not compensated for the services she provided.

While the violence that Mei suffered during the pandemic was not unique, as emerging research shows (Dietzel & Towfigh, 2023). Mei's situation exposes how the COVID-19 pandemic intensified the harm and challenges that marginalized students experience during their post-secondary education.

Black Lives Matter: Navigating COVID-19 and Systemic Racism

While the general population has struggled to cope with the uncertainty brought about by the pandemic, Black people have lived with daily uncertainties that threaten their lives. Dion asserted that Black people have experienced "two pandemics" in the forms of COVID-19 and systemic racism, since their lives have been endangered by the novel coronavirus and various forms of anti-Black violence. Specifically, Dion talked about how she felt negative psychological and emotional impacts related both to COVID-19 and witnessing the murders of George Floyd and Breonna Taylor in 2020, all of which "definitely played a part" in her overall health.

It is important to note that due to systemic inequities in society, which are exacerbated by the social determinants of health, Black populations are at a greater risk of being negatively impacted by COVID-19. In addition to experiencing higher rates of infection and death (CDC, 2021a), the pandemic has disproportionately impacted other aspects of Black people's lives, including the workplace, as people in equity seeking groups are overrepresented in essential workplaces. Due to economic turmoil Black people have suffered due to wealth and income disparities. Black people and racialized groups have also been burdened by the experience and stress of racial discrimination that has been shown to have negative effects on physical and mental health (CDC, 2021b). Black students were already experiencing racism and other barriers in their post-secondary education prior to the pandemic, such as being unfairly targeted by universities, anti-Black racism on campuses, and the many barriers to getting to a post-secondary campus in the first place (CBC, 2021; Maynard, 2017; Verma, 2018). Other research suggests that these issues may have worsened during the pandemic (Laurencin et al., 2020). In these ways, the COVID-19 pandemic exacerbated problems for already marginalized communities of Black students.

In response to the events surrounding the murders of George Floyd and Breonna Taylor in 2020, many post-secondary institutions in Canada released statements addressing anti-Black racism and systemic inequality. For example, the University of Windsor established initiatives to dismantle systemic practices and appointed a Black Student Support Coordinator to enhance support for Black students (University of Windsor, 2021). Additionally, the University of North Carolina at Chapel Hill's Department of Classics condemned these acts of violence and emphasized their commitment to social justice by taking actionable steps towards equity and inclusion within their department (University of North Carolina at Chapel Hill, 2020). While Dion's college provided information about the pandemic, her institution's response to the Black Lives Matter movement was non-existent: "I felt like [Black Lives Matter] was something that the college could have acknowledged. I didn't see anything. And they still haven't acknowledged it. This was very upsetting for me." As a Black student, Dion was disheartened by her institution's inaction: "It just got to a point where I just didn't want to do school." Similarly speaking to the difficulties of being a Black student in academia during the COVID-19 pandemic, Price (2020) wrote, "Black people have known crisis ever since the trans-Atlantic slave trade, and we have known it in the academy well before COVID-19. To be Black and active in the academy is to know what it means to survive, largely by practising what York University humanities scholar Christina Sharpe has termed 'care'" (para 11) (Sharpe, 2018). Price (2020) can be demonstrated by sharing information and resources on mental health for Black students, as well as space and time for Black students to connect with others on well-being. As mentioned, many academic institutions made statements and swiftly implemented initiatives to improve support for Black students, which can also be seen as acts of care. The absence of care for Black students and the lack of attention to anti-black racism demonstrated by the institution Dion attended created a sense of exclusion and a disinterest in her studies. Price (2020) also powerfully asserted that systemic racism "can be characterized as an enduring crisis, one that will most likely outlive our current pandemic" (para 4). During this time, Black students experienced threats to their safety and health from the COVID-19 pandemic and systemic racism, and Dion's testimonial highlights how post-secondary institutions can and must do more to support Black students and maintain a safe learning environment for them.

Although Dion could not "focus, concentrate and give my all in classes" and was struggling to deal with the COVID-19 pandemic and anti-Black racism, one of her professors denied a request she made for academic accommodations. Dion explained: "I felt like she should have understood that as a Black female, I am facing so many different things and still trying to be on top of my work. But the fact is that she was so unwilling to help in any way." The lack of support Dion received from her professor compounded the anxiety and stress she was already dealing with: "I just wanted to lay in bed and not think about everything that was happening. I was like, already over the class. I was over school." Overall, Dion's experience is an example of the "two pandemics" that she and other Black students were facing during the spring and summer of 2020. More research is urgently needed to understand how post-secondary institutions can improve their systems and better support Black students during times of crisis.

Indigenous Sovereignty & Covid-19

Indigenous Peoples in Canada also dealt with multiple, intersecting crises during the COVID-19 pandemic. In early 2020, international solidarity movements were mobilizing in support of the Wet'suwet'en whose lands were being invaded by Canada. Responding to the call from the Wet'suwet'en to "Shut down Canada", people demonstrated solidarity through ongoing blockades that pressured the government and targeted action from various industries (Unist'ot'en Camp, 2020).

Garrett said that, prior to March 2020, "railroads were shut down, the shipyards were stopped, and we had Wet'suwet'en protests going on across Canada. Then the pandemic happened."

Unfortunately, as Garrett explained, COVID-19 "overshadowed" movements for Indigenous sovereignty as the pandemic shifted focus away from the struggles of Indigenous Peoples and toward issues of public health and safety. Garrett also noted that Wet'suwet'en sovereign territory continues to be invaded by the state, as Canada aims to dispossess the Wet'suwet'en from their land. Specifically, Garrett was referencing an ongoing battle in British Columbia between Indigenous Peoples and the Royal Canadian Mounted Police (RCMP). Wet'suwet'en Hereditary Chiefs have been opposing the Coastal GasLink pipeline, calling for the police to get off their land but, despite these efforts, the RCMP has conducted militarized raids and patrolled Wet'suwet'en land (Hosgood, 2021a). At the time of writing this chapter, the fight between Wet'suwet'en and the RCMP continues, and a Hereditary Chief, Dsta'hyl from the Likhts'amisyu Clan was recently arrested for protesting the government's occupation of Indigenous territory (Hosgood, 2021b). Dsta'hyl is the first individual in Canada to be recognized as a prisoner of conscience by Amnesty International (Amnesty International, 2020). In July 2024, a Supreme Court Justice imposed a sentence of house arrest on Dsta'hyl, requiring him to remain at his home in Witset, a Wet'suwet'en community located approximately 700 kilometres north of Vancouver (CBC, 2024).

Importantly, Garrett drew parallels between Black people and Indigenous Peoples, linking their struggles against a common oppressor and citing shared histories of "colonization, slavery, and genocide". The needs of Black people and Indigenous Peoples have been ignored by the Canadian government (Canadian Human Rights Commission, 2021; Truth and Reconciliation Commission of Canada, 2015), and, in many cases, worsened by actions and inactions from the state (Canadian Human Rights Commission, 2020; Ontario Human Rights Commission, 2018a). Post-secondary educational institutions have also failed their Black and Indigenous students in many ways, perpetuating settler colonialism and white supremacy (Dei, 2012; Bhopal & Preston, 2012; Tuck & Yang, 2012). It is also important to note here that, like Black people, Indigenous Peoples are also at disproportionate risk of contracting COVID-19 (Sullivan et al., 2020). Garrett's experiences illuminate the connections between white supremacy and settler colonialism and the experiences of Black and Indigenous students during the pandemic. For these students, the challenges related to their identities and COVID-19 are interconnected and intensified by systemic inequities and injustices.

Garrett emphasized that, in addition to living through a global pandemic, Black people and Indigenous Peoples are threatened by law enforcement, who "should be helping and supporting marginalized communities". In fact, a recent report from the Council of Canadian Academies (2019) found that it is more than ten times more likely for Indigenous Peoples in Canada to be shot and killed by a police officer than white people. The COVID-19 pandemic has worsened existing disparities for marginalized communities, especially Black and Indigenous populations. High rates of police violence have continued during this time, with Black individuals in Toronto experiencing an arrest and lethal violence rate of 7.29 per million, higher than the U.S. average (Ontario Human Rights Commission, 2018b). As Sullivan et al. (2020) note, the pandemic has intensified the stressors of police brutality, leading to widespread vicarious trauma and significant physical, psychological, and educational harms. This highlights how the pandemic not only exacerbated inequities but also underscored the urgent need to address systemic injustices impacting these communities.

Dion's and Garrett's experiences show some of the ways in which the COVID-19 pandemic negatively impacted Black and Indigenous students' lives and their education. In reference to this, Dion stated that it was a "fear of all of these elements" that caused her to feel debilitated, without the capacity to engage in her studies. While interventions are urgently needed to address the cumulative and compounding effects of historic and ongoing racial injustice as well as the problems exacerbated by the COVID-19 pandemic, Dion's and Garrett's experiences remind us that the unpredictability and uncertainty brought about by the pandemic are not new, as Black and Indigenous students constantly deal with systemic oppression and marginalization in post-secondary institutions.

Dion's and Garrett's experiences underscore the urgent need for systemic change within post-secondary institutions. Their stories highlight the interplay between the ongoing challenges of racial injustice and the specific disruptions caused by the COVID-19 pandemic. Addressing these issues is critical not only for supporting Black and Indigenous students but also for fostering an equitable educational environment. As we move forward, we must acknowledge that the roots of these struggles run deep, necessitating sustained efforts to dismantle the barriers that continue to impede the success of marginalized communities.

Conclusion

The COVID-19 pandemic has impacted society in numerous ways, many of which we are just beginning to uncover. The findings from this chapter offer important insight into the experiences of marginalized post-secondary students, notably how the pandemic has exacerbated barriers that negatively impact these students' education. While our participants confronted these barriers in different ways, their experiences illustrate how historic oppressions factor into how they directly or indirectly experience current injustices. Some of oppressions examined in this chapter include racism and public institutions' responses to racism, colonialism and its lasting effects, and sexual violence. The experiences of students in this study suggest that systemic inequities may have been as impactful as the COVID-19 pandemic.

Participants' stories also showed that none of their experiences can be neatly carved off and contained; they are intimately intertwined. While it is easy to interpret these experiences as novel, we argue that the inequities related to the pandemic are an extension and exacerbation of pre-existing patterns. In Canada, marginalized students' post-secondary success is influenced by white supremacy, neo-colonial structures, and heteropatriarchal systems that seek to undermine, limit, and impair their potential. The rippling out of social inequities cannot be excused as happenstance; rather, they are woven into and reflect deep and sustained patterns of violence and oppression endemic to Canadian society.

The themes discussed in this chapter align with other emerging research in this field, which has shown that "COVID-19 is not the 'great equalizer' that some initially hailed it to be; instead, those already most marginalized will bear the brunt of suffering as the pandemic amplifies disparities created and sustained through structural inequities" (Sullivan et al., 2020, p. 28). Instead, students experiencing interlocking forms of marginalization, such as gender and race, as well as Indigenous and Black students, have experienced significantly more disruption to their studies (Music, 2020). The pandemic has brought social and racial injustice and inequity to the forefront of public discussion, and more work is urgently needed to address the legacies of oppression that exist in Canadian society and in post-secondary educational institutions.

Throughout this chapter, we have heard some of the many ways that students struggle, as well as how larger systemic issues are impacting their studies and university experiences. Post-secondary institutions need to adapt in meaningful ways that would support greater levels of success for marginalized students, particularly in crisis situations where pre-existing structural inequalities will inevitably come into play. As Swail (2014) said, "when an institution accepts the registration of a student, they are, in effect, entering a moral, ethical, and legal contract with the student to do whatever they can to help that student succeed" (p. 23). We argue that institutions can do better by taking a holistic view of student's well-being, which includes acknowledging students are human beings with lives and obligations outside of the classroom. We can better support students by prioritizing equity and justice, for example, by making anti-racist policies a priority. Doing so will help individuals and colonial structures – such as post-secondary institutions – work towards meaningful reconciliation. One of the first tangible steps toward accomplishing this goal is enacting and following through with the

Truth and Reconciliation Commission of Canada's (2015) 94 "Calls to Action". Among other things, we hope that this research can be part of informing meaningful change in post-secondary education.

An equitable learning environment both acknowledges and challenges the systemic, institutional, and interpersonal harm absorbed by marginalized students. During the pandemic, the needs of participants in this study were overlooked by their institutions, needs which are interlocking and build upon each other in ways that ripple out and have various impacts on their lives and education. These students matter, their struggles matter, and their success matters. We must continue telling the stories of marginalized students, sharing, and amplifying their messages as they battle their way through the COVID-19 pandemic and, as Price (2020) asserted, the "enduring crisis" of systemic oppression.

Limitations

Some study limitations should be acknowledged. The sample size for this study was small, limiting the generalizability of the sample. Future research can reconfirm study findings using larger scale studies.

References

Amnesty International. (2022). *Dsta'hyl: Canada's first prisoner of conscience*. Retrieved from Amnesty International. https://amnesty.ca/human-rights-news/canada-prisoner-of-conscience-completes-sentence/

Banerjee, D., & Rai, M. (2020). Social isolation in Covid-19: The impact of loneliness. *International Journal of Social Psychiatry, 66*(6), 525–527.

BC Centre for Disease Control. (2020). Distribution for illicit overdose deaths. Ministry of Public Safety and Solicitor General. https://www2.gov.bc.ca/assets/gov/birth-adoption-death-marriage-and-divorce/deaths/coroners-service/statistical/illicit-drug.pdf

Benhamou, K., & Piedra, A. (2020). CBT-informed interventions for essential workers during the COVID-19 pandemic. *Journal of Contemporary Psychotherapy, 50*(4), 275–283. https://doi.org/10.1007/s10879-020-09467-3

Bhopal, K., & Preston, J. (2012). *A systematic review of the literature on race and ethnicity in higher education in the UK. Journal of Educational Administration and History*, 44(1), 37–61. https://doi.org/10.1080/00220620.2011.613546

Brennan, S. (2011). Violent victimization of aboriginal women in the Canadian provinces, 2009 (Catalogue No. 85-02-X). Canadian Centre for Justice Statistics, Ministry of Industry. https://www150.statcan.gc.ca/n1/pub/85-002-x/2011001/article/11439-eng.pdf

Bricker, D. (2020). Majority (54%) of Canadians say physical distancing has left them feeling lonely or isolated. Ipsos. https://www.ipsos.com/en-ca/news-and-polls/Majority-Of-Canadians-Say-Physical-Distancing-Has-Left-Them-Feeling-Lonely-Or-Isolated

British Columbia. (2020, October 21). Virtual mental health supports during COVID-19. *Mental Health and Substance Use.* https://www2.gov.bc.ca/gov/content/health/managing-your-health/mental-health-substance-use/virtual-mental-health-supports

Burke, B., & Harrison, P. (1998). Anti-oppressive practice. In J. Dalrymple (Ed.), *Anti-oppressive social work practice* (pp. 229–239). Palgrave.

Canadian Association of University Teachers. (2020). *Racism and the university: Addressing systemic racism in higher education.* Retrieved from https://www.caut.ca

Canadian Broadcasting Corporation. (2021). Being Black on campus: Why students, staff and faculty say universities are failing them. *The Fifth Estate.* https://www.cbc.ca/news/canada/anti-black-racism-campus-university-1.5924548

Canadian Broadcasting Corporation News. (2024, July 31). *Amnesty International recognizes Dsta'hyl as Canada's first prisoner of conscience.* https://www.cbc.ca/news/canada/british-columbia/amnesty-international-prisoner-of-conscience-1.7280904

Canadian Human Rights Commission. (2020). *Federal government response to the COVID-19 pandemic: Impact on Indigenous peoples.* Retrieved from https://www.chrc-ccdp.gc.ca/eng/content/federal-government-response-covid-19-pandemic-impact-indigenous-peoples

Canadian Human Rights Commission (2021). *Anti-Racism Action Plan: Progress Report June 1, 2021.* https://www.chrc-ccdp.gc.ca/resources/publications/anti-racism-action-plan-progress-report-june-1-2021

Canadian Women's Foundation. (2021). The facts about sexual assault and harassment. https://canadianwomen.org/the-facts/sexual-assault-harassment/

Centers for Disease Control and Prevention. (2021a). Risk for COVID-19 infection, hospitalization, and death by race/ethnicity. https://www.cdc.gov/coronavirus/2019-ncov/covid-data/investigations-discovery/hospitalization-death-by-race-ethnicity.html

Centers for Disease Control and Prevention. (2021b). Health equity considerations and racial and ethnic minority groups, *COVID-19.* https://www.cdc.gov/coronavirus/2019-ncov/community/health-equity/race-ethnicity.html

Christoffersen, A., & Emejulu, A. (2023). "Diversity Within": The Problems with "Intersectional" White Feminism in Practice. *Social Politics: International Studies in Gender, State & Society, 30*(2), 630–653. https://doi.org/10.1093/sp/jxac044

Collins, P. H. (2000). *Black feminist thought: Knowledge, consciousness, and the politics of empowerment.* Routledge.

Cotter, A. (2018). Intimate partner violence: Experiences of visible minority women in Canada, 2018. *Statistics Canada.* https://www150.statcan.gc.ca/n1/pub/85-002-x/2021001/article/00008-eng.htm

Crenshaw, K. (1989). Demarginalizing the intersection of race and sex: A black feminist critique of antidiscrimination doctrine, feminist theory, and antiracist politics. *University of Chicago Legal Forum, 1989*(1), 139–167.

Crenshaw, K. (1990). Mapping the margins: Intersectionality, identity politics, and violence against women of color. *Stanford Law Review, 43*(6), 1241–1299.

Crenshaw, K. (2017). *On intersectionality: Essential writings.* The New Press.

Crosby, S. [@themindgeek] (n.d.). Instagram. Retrieved November 8, 2021, from https://www.instagram.com/themindgeek/?hl=en

Dei, G. J. S. (2012). *Indigenous knowledge and education: A transformative framework.* In *Indigenous education and the role of educators* (pp. 17–29). Springer.

Dietzel, C., & Towfigh, K. (Eds.). (2024). *Pandemic injustice: Navigating legal and policy lines during the COVID-19 pandemic.* Confronting systemic omissions and impacts in educational policy. First edition. New York, NY: Peter Lang.

Dominelli, L. (2002). *Anti-oppressive social work theory and practice.* Palgrave Macmillan.

Foundry [@foundry_bc] (n.d.). Instagram. Retrieved November 8, 2021, from https://www.instagram.com/foundry_bc/?hl=en

Government of Canada. (2021). *Indigenous services: Key facts about First Nations, Métis, and Inuit.* Retrieved from https://www.sac-isc.gc.ca/eng/1506511377383/1535072079387

Gupta, R., & Ariefdjohan, M. (2021). Mental illness on Instagram: A mixed method study to characterize public content, sentiments, and trends of antidepressant use. *Journal of Mental Health, 30*(4), 518–525.

hooks, b. (2000). *Where we stand: Class matters.*

Hosgood, A. F. (2021, August 16). RCMP has spent almost $20 million policing Wet'suwet'en Territory. *The Tyee.* https://thetyee.ca/News/2021/08/16/RCMP-Spent-Almost-20-Million-Policing-Wetsuweten-Territory/

Hosgood, A. F. (2021, October 29). Arrest of Wet'suwet'en Hereditary Chief 'So Insulting'. *The Tyee.* https://thetyee.ca/News/2021/10/29/Arrest-Wetsuweten-Hereditary-Chief-So-Insulting/

Jones, A., Smith, B., & Nguyen, C. (2021). Impact of COVID-19 on marginalized college students. *Journal of Higher Education Research, 34*(2), 150–165.

Kaniasty, K., Moore, K. A., Howard, S., & Buchwald, P. (Eds.). (2014). *Stress and anxiety: Applications to social and environmental threats, psychological well-being, occupational challenges, and developmental psychology.* Logos Verlag Berlin GmbH.

Kemp, S. (2020). Digital 2020: July global statshot. *DATAREPORTAL.* https://datareportal.com/reports/digital-2020-july-global-statshot

Lavrakas, P. (2008). Convenience sampling. *Encyclopedia of Survey Research Methods.* https://dx.doi.org/10.4135/9781412963947.n105

Laurencin, C. T., & Walker, J. M. (2020). A pandemic on a pandemic: Racism and COVID-19 in Blacks. *Cell Systems, 11*(1), 9–10. https://doi.org/10.1016/j.cels.2020.07.002

Logie, C., Alaggia, R., & Rwigema, M. (2017). A social ecological approach to understanding correlates of lifetime sexual assault among sexual minority women in Toronto, Canada: Results from a cross-sectional internet-based survey, *Health Education Research, 29*(4), 671–682, https://doi.org/10.1093/her/cyt119.

Mackenzie, C., & Fagan, R. (2018). *Anti-oppressive practice in social work: A critical reflection on the impact of the social work profession. Social Work Education*, 37(4), 459–472. https://doi.org/10.1080/02615479.2018.1437341

Mansbridge, J. J., & Morris, A. (Eds.). (2001). *Oppositional consciousness: The subjective roots of social protest.* University of Chicago Press.

Maynard, R. (2017). Canadian education is steeped in anti-Black racism. *The Walrus.* https://thewalrus.ca/canadian-education-is-steeped-in-anti-black-racism/

Mental Health Commission of Canada. (2012). Changing directions changing lives. *The Mental Health Strategy for Canada, 80*(4) 78–92. https://www.mentalhealthcommission.ca/wp-content/uploads/drupal/MHStrategy_Strategy_ENG.pdf

Michigan Medicine. (2023). *Mental health concerns among university students: 2023 survey results.* Retrieved from https://caps.umich.edu/article/u-m-college-student-mental-health-survey-phase-v.

Michalski, J., Cunningham, T., & Henry, J. (2017). The diversity challenge for higher education in Canada. *Digital Commons, Humboldt State University.* https://digitalcommons.humboldt.edu/cgi/viewcontent.cgi?

Music, G. (2020). COVID, racism and Black lives matter: A deadly constellation. *Developmental Child Welfare, 2*(3), 197–207.

Ontario Human Rights Commission. (2018a). A collective impact: Interim report on the inquiry into racial profiling and racial discrimination of Black persons by the Toronto Police Service, *Ontario Human Rights Commission Interim Report.* http://www.ohrc.on.ca/sites/default/files/TPS%20Inquiry_Interim%20Report%20EN%20FINAL%20DESIGNED%20for%20remed_3_0.pdf#overlay-context=en/news_centre/ohrc-interim-report-toronto-police-service-inquiry-shows-disturbing-results

Ontario Human Rights Commission. (2018b). *A time for action: Addressing anti-Black racism in Ontario.* Retrieved from http://www.ohrc.on.ca/en/report-time-action-addressing-anti-black-racism-ontario

Peterman, A., Potts, A., O'Donnell, M., Thompson, K., Shah, M., Oertwig, P., & O'Leary, C. (2020). *Pandemic domestic violence: The impact of COVID-19 on intimate partner violence and the need for response.* World Bank. Retrieved from https://openknowledge.worldbank.org

Patel, R. (2020). Minister says COVID-19 is empowering domestic violence abusers as rates rise in parts of Canada, *Canadian Broadcasting Corporation.* https://www.cbc.ca/news/politics/domestic-violence-rates-rising-due-to-covid19-1.5545851

Price, N. (2020, July 19). Addressing anti-Black racism in post-secondary institutions can transform Canada after the COVID-19 pandemic. *The Conversation.* https://theconversation.com/addressing-anti-black-racism-in-post-secondary-institutions-can-transform-canada-after-the-covid-19-pandemic-141366

Reetz, D. R., Krylowicz, B., & Mistler, B. (2014). *The Association for University and College Counseling Center Directors Annual Survey, 2013–2014.* AUCCCD. https://www.aucccd.org/assets/documents/2014%20aucccd%20monograph%20-%20public%20pdf.pdf

Sanders, T & Hardy, K. (2015). Students selling sex: Marketisation, higher education and consumption. *British Journal of Sociology of Education, 36*(5), 747–765.

Scrim, K. (2017). Victims of crime research No. 3: Aboriginal victimization in Canada: A summary of the literature. https://www.justice.gc.ca/eng/rp-pr/cj-jp/victim/rd3-rr3/p3.html#sec3

Sharpe, C. (2018). *And to survive. Small Axe*, 22(3), 171–178. https://doi.org/10.1215/17932192-7315267

Sinacore, A. L., Jaghori, B., & Rezazadeh, M. S. (2014). Female university students working in the sex trade: A narrative analysis. *Canadian Journal of Counselling and Psychotherapy, 49*(1), 40–56.

Statistics Canada. (2016). Leading causes of death, total population, by age group, Canada, 2016 (Table 13-10-0394-01). Retrieved from https://www150.statcan.gc.ca/t1/tbl1/en/tv.action?pid=1310039401

Statistics Canada. (2011). Measuring violence against women: Statistical trends: highlights. https://www150.statcan.gc.ca/n1/pub/85-002-x/2013001/article/11766-eng.htm

Statistics Canada. (2020a). Mental health of Canadians during the COVID-19 pandemic. https://www150.statcan.gc.ca/n1/pub/11-627-m/11-627-m2020039-eng.htm

Statistics Canada. (2020b). Confirmed cases of COVID-19. https://www.sac-isc.gc.ca/eng/1598625105013/1598625167707

Statistics Canada. (2020c). How are postsecondary students in Canada impacted by the COVID-19 pandemic? https://www150.statcan.gc.ca/n1/pub/11-627-m/ 11-627-m2020032-eng.htm

Statistics Canada. (2020d). *Impacts of COVID-19 on post-secondary students.* Retrieved from https://www.statcan.gc.ca/en/subjects-start/covid-19

Statistics Canada. (2020e). *Canadian post-secondary students and the COVID-19 pandemic: Survey results.* Retrieved from https://www.statcan.gc.ca/en/subjects-start/covid-19

Sullivan, A., Miller, F. G., McKevvett, N. M., Muldrew, A., Hansen-Burke, A. & Weeks, M. (2020). Leveraging MTSS to advance, not suppress COVID-related equity issues. *Communique, 49*(1), 1–29.

Swail, W. (2014). A different viewpoint on student retention. *Higher Learning Research Communications.* https://files.eric.ed.gov/fulltext/EJ1133252.pdf

Takeuchi, C. (2020). Vancouver police arrest 46 people who refused to leave CRAB Park encampment. *The Georgia Straight.* https://www.straight.com/news/vancouver-police-force-homeless-campers-to-relocate-from-crab-park

Tang, J., Galbraith, N., & Truong, J. (2019). Living alone in Canada: Insights on Canadian society. Statistics Canada. https://www150.statcan.gc.ca/n1/pub/75-006-x/2019001/article/00003-eng.htm

The Council for Canadian Academies. (2019). Toward peace, harmony, and well-being: Policing in Indigenous communities. The Expert Panel on Policing in Indigenous Communities. https://cca-reports.ca/wp-content/uploads/2019/04/FullReport-Toward-Peace-Harmony-and-WellBeing.pdf

The Daily. (2020). Impact of the COVID-19 pandemic on postsecondary students, *Statistics Canada.* https://www150.statcan.gc.ca/n1/en/daily-quotidien/200512/dq200512a-eng.pdf?st=0nOLRxKr

Torres, C. A. (2017). *Decolonizing knowledge: The role of knowledge in the process of decolonization.* In *Decolonization and the Ethics of Research* (pp. 55–75).

Torres N. M. (2017). Fanon and decolonial thought. In M. A. Peters (Ed.) *Encyclopedia of educational philosophy and theory.* Springer. https://doi.org/10.1007/978-981-287-588-4_506

Truth and Reconciliation Commission of Canada. (2015). Calls to Action. https://www2.gov.bc.ca/assets/gov/british-columbians-our-governments/indigenous-people/aboriginal-peoples-documents/calls_to_action_english2.pdf

Truth and Reconciliation Commission of Canada. (2015). *Honouring the truth, reconciling for the future: Summary of the final report of the Truth and Reconciliation Commission of Canada.* Retrieved from http://nctr.ca/assets/reports/Final%20Reports/Executive_Summary_English_Web.pdf

Tuck, E., & Yang, K. W. (2012). *Decolonization is not a metaphor. Decolonization: Indigeneity, Education & Society*, 1(1), 1–40. Retrieved from https://decolonization.org/index.php/des/article/view/18630

UN Women. (2020). *The shadow pandemic: Violence against women during COVID-19.* Retrieved from https://www.unwomen.org

UN Women. (2021). COVID-19 and ending violence against women and girls, *United Nations Entity for Gender Equality and the Empowerment of Women (UN Women).* https://www.unwomen.org/en/digital-library/publications/2020/04/issue-brief-covid-19-and-ending-violence-against-women-and-girls

Unist'ot'en Camp. (2020). *All eyes on Wet'suwet'en: International call for solidarity!* https://unistoten.camp/alleyesonwetsuweten/

University of North Carolina at Chapel Hill. (2020). *Department of Classics condemns violence against Black lives.* Retrieved from https://classics.unc.edu

University of Windsor. (2021). *Anti-Black racism initiatives and support for Black students.* Retrieved from https://www.uwindsor.ca/anti-black-racism

Verma, S. (2018). Black students still face major hurdles getting into university. *McMaster News, McMaster University.* https://brighterworld.mcmaster.ca/articles/black-students-still-face-major-hurdles-getting-into-university/

Watson, B. (2020, March 30). How one lonely clapper in Vancouver's West End sparked the 7 p.m. health-care workers salute. *Canadian Broadcasting Corporation.* https://www.cbc.ca/news/canada/british-columbia/rory-richards-applause-healthcare-workers-1.5515099

World Health Organization. (2021). *Addressing violence against women in the context of the COVID-19 pandemic.* Retrieved from https://www.who.int

· 3 ·

BETWEEN THE ROCK AND THE HARD PLACE: EXPLORING THE EFFECTS OF COVID-19 ON ONE STUDENT'S MENTAL WELL-BEING IN ENGLAND USING THE AUTO-HERMENEUTIC APPROACH

Zineb Boudiba

The COVID-19 pandemic has profoundly impacted not only the social lives of individuals but also their psychological well-being. This chapter examines the effects of the pandemic on my experience as an international student in the United Kingdom (UK), contextualized within a review of fourteen studies exploring the pandemic's impact on university students in the UK, the USA and Canada. Employing an auto-hermeneutic approach, the study interprets my personal experience as a PhD international student in the UK. Key findings from both the literature review and the auto-hermeneutic analysis reveal that loneliness, concerns for family members, a loss of direction, academic uncertainty, reduced physical activity and socioeconomic challenges were prevalent psychological stressors. The study makes two primary contributions to the literature. First, it adopts an interactionist approach to analyse how contextual factors influence individual experiences, particularly highlighting the role of internal motivators in mitigating the effects of external adversities on well-being. Second, it extends the application of auto-hermeneutics, a methodology traditionally associated with information processing sciences, to the field of health sciences. Additionally, this research enriches the discourse on resilience by illuminating the role of faith in fostering a resilient mindset during periods of crisis. By integrating personal narrative with empirical analysis, the study offers a nuanced understanding of the psychological challenges faced by international students during the pandemic and the strategies employed to navigate such adversities.

The COVID-19 pandemic has had profound implications not only for the physical health of global populations, including general health deteriorations, but also for their mental well-being. The World Health Organization (WHO, 2026) defines mental health as "a state of mental well-being that enables people to cope with the stresses of life, realize their abilities, learn and work well, and contribute to their community" (Concepts in Mental Health section). In this research, I adopt the definition proposed by Galderisi et al. (2015), as it emphasizes the capacity to regulate emotions in the face of adversity, aligning closely with the objectives of this study. According to Galderisi et al. (2015, p. 232), mental health is "a dynamic state of internal equilibrium which enables individuals to use their abilities in harmony with universal values of society". This includes basic cognitive and social skills, the ability to recognize, express and modulate one's emotions, empathy, flexibility in coping with adverse life events, functioning in social roles and maintaining a harmonious relationship between body and mind. These components collectively contribute to an individual's internal equilibrium.

In response to the rapid spread of COVID-19, the United Kingdom implemented its first national lockdown on 23 March 2020 (Zhou & Kan, 2021). The containment measures, including self-isolation, significantly disrupted the normal trajectories of individuals' lives (The UK Parliament Office of Science and Technology, 2021). In the academic sector, universities transitioned from face-to-face instruction to online learning as part of social distancing protocols (Zavlis et al., 2021). Research on tertiary-level students in the UK has highlighted the adverse effects of the pandemic on their mental well-being. For instance, the Office for National Statistics (2020) reported that 58 % of students experienced a decline in their mental health due to COVID-19. These findings underscore the negative impact of the pandemic on the student population in the UK.

The mental well-being of PhD students has been a growing area of research, particularly in light of the unique challenges they faced during COVID-19, such as academic pressure, financial strain and social isolation. Pyhältö et al. (2023) explored the pandemic's impact on 768 PhD candidates in Finland. Their mixed-method study revealed that international students faced unique vulnerabilities, namely an increased isolation, academic challenges and financial strain. Similar findings were reported in a cross-sectional study conducted by Evans et al. (2021), which surveyed 297 doctoral students in the United States. They identified that well-being during the pandemic was influenced by emotional connections to loved ones and coping mechanisms. Participants primarily relied on emotional support from loved ones and peers, alongside self-care practices like physical exercise, meditation and praying and seeking professional help, to manage stress and anxiety.

Similarly, Sverdlik et al. (2022) identified that social isolation, exacerbated by the inability to connect with family and friends, significantly worsened mental health among 708 international doctoral students across various countries (USA, UK, Canada, Australia, Asia and the Middle East). This was compounded by academic challenges, particularly for students dependent on fieldwork or in-person interactions, which raised concerns about research. The academic concerns faced by PhD students during the COVID-19 pandemic align with the findings of Aristeidou and Aristidou (2023), whose study specifically examined the experiences of 1,780 PhD students in the UK during this period. Their study highlighted the significant impact of personal circumstances (e.g. caring responsibilities) and financial concerns on mental health. Students without funded extensions were more likely to experience depression, underscoring the role of financial stability in mental well-being. Collectively, these factors contributed to heightened levels of stress and exhaustion among PhD students.

Most studies examining the effects of the pandemic on students' mental health have employed quantitative research designs, utilizing cross-sectional online surveys (e.g. Catling et al., 2022; Lai et al., 2020; McGivern & Shepherd, 2022; Office for National Statistics, 2020). In contrast, fewer studies have adopted qualitative methodologies (e.g. Burns et al., 2020). Notably, no research to date has utilized an auto-hermeneutic approach to explore the pandemic's impact on international students, enabling them to reflect on and interpret their own experiences. This chapter addresses this gap by introducing the unique potential of auto-hermeneutics to uncover insights that other methods may overlook, such as the role of faith in mental well-being. Furthermore, auto-hermeneutics is particularly suited to this study due to its focus on understanding the relationship between individuals and their world. Drawing on Merleau-Ponty's hermeneutic philosophy, which emphasizes the person–world relationship (Smith & Nizza, 2022), auto-hermeneutics examines personal experiences to elucidate how the world shapes individuals' beliefs, perceptions and behaviours.

This study seeks to address the following research questions: (1) What was the impact of COVID-19 on the mental health of one international student? (2) How did one international student cope with the stress induced by COVID-19? and (3) To what extent do the findings from the experience of one international student align with the existing literature on the impact of COVID-19 on international students?

The chapter is structured as follows: the methodology section provides a detailed explanation of the auto-hermeneutic approach and the narrative review.

The findings section presents an analysis and interpretation of my personal experience, utilizing core and post-experience reflections (Gorichanaz, 2017), and situates these insights within the context of the narrative review. The discussion section concludes the chapter by highlighting the strengths and limitations of the study, as well as offering recommendations for future research.

Methodology

This section provides a detailed explanation of the two methods employed in this study for data collection and analysis: the auto-hermeneutic approach and narrative review.

The Auto-Hermeneutic Approach

Auto-hermeneutics involves the study of the self, examining individuals' perceptions, emotions and experiences to understand a phenomenon within its broader context (Gorichanaz, 2017). A key advantage of this approach lies in its potential to enrich others' lives by fostering reflection and empathy through the presentation of personal narratives. By engaging with cultural or social accounts of individual experiences, readers may encounter previously unconsidered realities, highlighting the value of self-study as a meaningful form of inquiry (Méndez-López, 2013). This methodology offers several strengths, including the generation of richly detailed insider perspectives and access to hidden or marginalized social worlds (Adams & Manning, 2015; Wall, 2008).

Examining one's own experiences yields intricate, layered insights that capture the depth and complexity of cultural phenomena. This method leverages privileged access to personal memories, emotions and embodied knowledge, enabling the reconstruction of vivid, multisensory accounts that immerse readers in the lived reality of the experience (Adams & Manning, 2015). Such an insider perspective reveals nuanced dimensions of cultural contexts often overlooked by external observers, providing a more authentic and comprehensive understanding of the phenomenon under study. This approach not only enriches academic discourse but also bridges gaps between diverse lived experiences, fostering greater empathy and awareness among readers.

Experience is both subjective and socially intersubjective, encompassing past and present dimensions (Caru & Cova, 2015; Ellway & Dean, 2016). In this study, intersubjectivity is evident in my reflections on the pandemic's impact on my mental well-being. Consequently, the interpretation of data gathered through the auto-hermeneutic approach was influenced by internal constructs such as beliefs and personality, which collectively constitute the self. External factors, including the pandemic, quarantine and academic pressures, represent the "other".

Data Collection for the Auto-Hermeneutic Approach

I recorded my thoughts and emotions during the first wave of the pandemic, from March 2020 to September 2020, resulting in four hours of audio recordings. Initially, these recordings were not intended for research purposes but served as a therapeutic tool to support my mental well-being during the pandemic. However, upon identifying a methodological gap in the literature on the effects of COVID-19 on university students, I repurposed these recordings as data. In 2022, I transcribed and translated the recordings into English. Despite their original intent, these recordings proved invaluable in capturing detailed descriptions of my emotions and coping mechanisms during the pandemic. I recorded myself in the Algerian Arabic dialect to facilitate free expression and later translated the content into English for analysis.

Narrative Review

A literature review is defined as a systematic methodology to identify current issues or future implications within a given subject (Grant & Booth, 2009). Reviewing and synthesizing findings from multiple studies helps identify gaps in existing research, generate new hypotheses and provide contextualization for new investigations (Kitchenham & Charters, 2007). In this study, the narrative review helped identify a methodological gap – specifically, the lack of phenomenological and hermeneutic studies on the impact of COVID-19 on individuals – as well as the under-representation of international students in research focused primarily on domestic students in the UK. Additionally, it facilitated the adoption of an interactionist approach to examine the pandemic's impact on students.

I selected a narrative review for two primary reasons: (1) to explore new perspectives and broaden the scope of the literature and (2) because the narrative review aligns with interpretivism, which reflects my epistemological stance in this research. The first reason is evident in the study's aim, which is not to generalize findings but to shed light on new insights regarding the pandemic's effects on international students in the UK. This objective aligns with the purpose of the narrative review, which does not seek to generalize findings (Green et al., 2006), and the auto-hermeneutic approach, which investigates new perspectives to expand the literature. The second reason for choosing a narrative review is its interpretative nature, which complements the auto-hermeneutic approach. A narrative review relies on the researcher's interpretation to generate or expand knowledge in a specific field (Green et al., 2006). In this study, this interpretation is manifested in the analysis of my experience as an international PhD student in the UK during the pandemic and how it aligns with the experiences of other students.

To address the three research questions, I conducted a thematic search for relevant studies using terms such as "the effects/impacts of COVID-19 on university students in the UK", which I later narrowed to focus on "international students in the UK". I also included a few studies from Canada and the USA, as they involved international students from the UK. From this search, I selected fourteen articles, classifying their findings according to the themes derived from the auto-hermeneutic recordings.

Findings

This section presents the findings derived from the auto-hermeneutic approach and the narrative review. The data collected through the auto-hermeneutic approach is organized into three subsections: setting, core-experience and post-experience. The setting does not refer to pre-experience, as the focus is on my experiences specifically during and after the pandemic, rather than before it. Instead, the setting describes the context in which the core and post-experiences occurred. Additionally, this section discusses the findings of the narrative review in relation to the auto-hermeneutic findings.

Setting

This subsection outlines the contextual factors that influenced my PhD journey in the UK during the COVID-19 pandemic. I was awarded a fully funded scholarship to pursue a PhD in the UK from 2020 to 2023. To address the research questions initially designed for my project, I planned to travel to Algeria in 2021 to conduct fieldwork and collect data. However, the rapid spread of COVID-19 led to the closure of international borders, including those of the UK and Algeria. The UK government advised against all non-essential global travel, while Algeria suspended marine and aviation transportation with Europe starting in March 2020. The UK officially announced its first lockdown in March 2020. The initial impact of the lockdown on my mental health stemmed from my inability to travel between the UK and Algeria for two years, as international travel only resumed in 2022.

My experience as an international student in the UK during the pandemic can be examined through two dimensions: academic and personal. This experience can be conceptualized as a cause–effect relationship, where the pandemic's impact on my PhD (academic) directly affected my mental health (personal). This interplay will be explored in greater detail in the core-experience section. The convergence of several factors – such as the time constraints of the PhD programme, the reduction of financial sponsorship and the suspension of flights between Algeria and the UK – represented significant external stressors during the lockdown period (2020–2022).

The shift to online data collection during the pandemic necessitated substantial changes to the focus, methodology and analysis of my PhD research. Within a year, I had to identify a new research topic, adapt the methodology and collect data remotely rather than in person. Initially, my PhD project aimed to investigate the educational policies of teacher education programmes from the perspectives of teacher trainers in Initial Teacher Education centres and novice teachers in special education schools in Algeria. However, due to the pandemic, the revised topic focused on the resilience of four special education teachers in Algeria, who were interviewed online. The following quote, recorded during my data collection period, illustrates the external factors that contributed to my mental well-being and were directly tied to my PhD. This excerpt also exemplifies how I vocalized my concerns during the pandemic to seek solutions, aligning with my use of audio recordings as a therapeutic coping mechanism:

> Now, with the closure of borders between Algeria and the UK, I can't go to Algeria and conduct my fieldwork. Even the Initial Teacher Education Centers are not responding to my calls and emails for the online interviews. Now I have only four participants, and I need to think quickly about how I can adjust this PhD and make something meaningful out of it; otherwise, I am doomed.

Core-Experience

The core-experience analysis identified three themes from the audio recordings: isolation during the pandemic, the use of religion as a coping mechanism and physical fitness exercises. These themes were analysed through an interactionist lens (person-world rapport) to understand the effects of external stressors on my mental well-being and how I employed internal motivators to cope. These themes were also compared with findings from the fourteen studies included in the narrative review to identify similarities and differences between my experience and those of other university students in the literature.

Isolation During COVID-19

The first significant impact of the pandemic on my mental well-being was evident in my disrupted sleep patterns and the onset of insomnia during the first lockdown in 2020. Insomnia, commonly defined as difficulty sleeping, is often associated with heightened stress levels (Roth, 2007). I categorized the factors contributing to my insomnia into two groups. First, academic–pandemic reasons, including the time constraints of the PhD programme, the reduction of financial sponsorship, and the closure of borders between Algeria and the UK. Second, individual-pandemic reasons, such as the death of family members due to COVID-19, self-isolation during the lockdown, and my own physical illness from COVID-19.

The interplay between academic and individual pandemic-related factors during the first and second lockdowns in 2020 shaped my perception of the pandemic's impact on my mental well-being as an international student in the UK. This dynamic can be explained as the outcome of my interaction with the world – specifically, how I responded to external factors beyond my control (e.g. the pandemic, family bereavement, financial instability and academic challenges). These factors collectively exhausted my mental health, as I had to navigate these adversities for nearly three years while striving to maintain a positive outlook. This tension between battling external challenges and sustaining internal resilience highlights how the interaction between external stressors and internal coping mechanisms contributes to stress and, consequently, affects mental health.

When analysing the data from the audio recordings, I identified one central individual-pandemic theme: isolation. Doing a PhD as an international student in the UK whilst self-isolating from March 2020 to March 2021 negatively affected my sleeping patterns. I developed insomnia for one year. To reduce the spread of the virus, the university cancelled workshops and Post-Graduate Research activities in which different PhD students had the opportunity to share their concerns and hold discussions. This cancellation reduced the chances for both home and international PhD students to meet and voice their academic issues and relate to each other. It resulted in an increased feeling of isolation caused by the quarantine as well as the pressure of the PhD. Therefore, the effect of *self-isolation* in this study on my mental well-being was caused by quarantining during the pandemic and the loneliness during a PhD, in addition to the intersection between the pandemic and my academic studies, which resulted in reshaping my initial PhD topic.

The following extract describes the beginning of the impact that the change from face-to-face to online delivery mode had on me. It highlights the effect of isolation on my academic life, which in turn negatively impacted my personal one. This quote again demonstrates how mental health is affected by the intertwinement between academic and personal factors.

> Now that everything is online, I can't even go to the library or the University or socialize like I used to. [Sighs] It will be so hard for me to study, sleep, relax, and eat in the same room. I hate spending all my time in one place. I will be suffocated, but it's okay I must adapt. There is no time for complaints.

The language used to describe this effect included "suffocated, oufff, hard for me" which indicated a state of discomfort that was caused by the external factor (i.e. regulations and measures to reduce the spread of COVID-19). The passage also indicated a willingness to comply with the sudden change whilst neglecting inner emotions, which were voiced through a feeling of complaint. This passage is significant because it reflects the struggle between personal preference to academic delivery mode, adaptation to sudden change and neglecting the feeling of being suffocated during the pandemic, which appeared through my feeling of loneliness and therefore affected my mental stability.

Isolation in the Narrative Review

The analysis from the previous passage is in accordance with the narrative review. A number of studies investigating the impact of the pandemic on international students reported that loneliness was a significant psychological factor that affected individuals' mental well-being (Appleby et al., 2022; Catling et al., 2022; Chen & Lucock, 2022; Maleku et al., 2022; McGivern & Shepherd, 2022). Among the psychological stressors expressed by international students, Maleku et al. (2022) put particular emphasis on discrimination, loneliness, anxiety and depression. Their review also revealed the impact of online teaching procedures on students' loneliness, which is similar to my findings from the auto-hermeneutic approach. Lai et al. (2020) compared the experiences of international students who returned to their home countries in Asia with the ones who stayed in their host countries (USA and UK). The findings indicate that depression among international students was associated with online delivery because their expectations at the beginning of the course were to socialize with other students. Therefore, loneliness and discrimination were among the leading causes of depression.

Within the same theme of loneliness, McGivern and Shepherd (2022) conducted a qualitative study using content analysis (CA) to analyse the experience of 82 students in northeast England. The findings were classified under three major themes: education, health and quality of life. Within the second theme (health), students reported a deterioration in both physical and mental health. Precisely, stress, anxiety, depression and loneliness were the prevailing symptoms reported by half of the participants (forty-three students) (McGivern & Shepherd, 2022). Regarding the quality of life, twenty-three participants reported lack of socialization and isolation affected their mental well-being because they affected their usual routine, which reduced their motivation towards their daily activities. Similarly, Appleby et al. (2022) compared the effects of COVID-19 on the mental health of students in the UK and Canada. The key findings indicated that social isolation and loneliness affected students' regular lifestyle (i.e. from face-to-face to online) in the UK and Canada and therefore, negatively impacted their mental well-being.

Within the theme of anxiety and depression, Catling et al. (2022) conducted a study on university students in the UK. The findings of this study revealed that the level of anxiety and depression rose among students, which made them addicted to their smartphones. This finding appeared to be affected by the level of loneliness the students experienced during the COVID-19 pandemic. It could be concluded that the studies mentioned above (Appleby et al., 2022; Burns et al., 2020; Catling et al., 2022; Lai et al., 2020; Maleku et al., 2022; McGivern & Shepherd, 2022) highlighted the same impact of the COVID-19 pandemic on the mental well-being of university students: anxiety, depression and loneliness. This finding is in line with the analysis from my auto-hermeneutic approach.

The Use of Religion to Maintain Psychological Well-Being

My concern about my family members marked the second aspect that impacted my mental well-being, specifically through insomnia and depression. It involved the death of several family members during the pandemic and my inability to attend their funerals. The emotional empathy towards others appeared to impact my psychological well-being, which was manifested through insomnia (a pattern of 2–3 hours of sleep per day for one year). Overall, each of these reasons was mutually influential to one another in the sense that the death of family members affected my insomnia because of self-isolation, and the suspended flights during the lockdown increased my depression during the pandemic. The interplay between these factors also reflects the influence of both external stressors (unexpected death, closed borders because of the pandemic) and personal factors (feeling isolated and insomnia) on mental well-being. This suggests that stable or shaken mental well-being could be a product of the interaction of individuals and what happens in the world surrounding them.

The following passage describes how I voiced my inner concerns, yet I comforted myself with the belief in Allah, who was by my side when facing external stressors.

> Oh okay, I know that the death rate is rising in Algeria. My Aunt and other family members passed away (may Allah have mercy on them and grant them paradise). I am unable to go and be with my family at this moment. Everything will be fine. I just need to have faith.

This excerpt also introduces another key finding in this study: the influence of religious beliefs on maintaining mental well-being during stressful times. To explain this construct, the religious belief that helped me protect my psychological stability during hard times was submitting to the will of Allah (God). This will include the belief that everything was destined to happen at that specific time (i.e. during the lockdown) and place (my presence in the UK and my family's location in Algeria).

Maintaining a resilient mindset during the pandemic was associated with my identity as a Muslim. Islamic values such as faith in the creator *Allah* (God) and the belief in destiny contributed to my mental strength. Faith in Islam is related to acceptance of destiny (*Redha* in Arabic) in order to reach a degree of piety (*taqwa* in Arabic). This religious internalization positively influenced my mindset and helped me cope with the stress of losing family members whilst being isolated in the UK. The following extract was recorded during the second lockdown (2021), precisely after I received the news about the deaths of my family members.

> I can't fly to Algeria. It is safe for me and my family to stay where I am. I don't want to catch COVID-19 on my way home from the airport and contaminate my family. Allah is my refuge: I entrust myself and my family to Allah as I belief nothing will happen to me or to my family with the will of Allah (Say: nothing will happen to us except what Allah has decreed for us: he is our protector). So, it is better for me to stay where I am.

In this quote, I referred to a verse from the Quran (Surat Al-tawba, verse 51) to remind myself that everything happening at the time was destined to happen. This belief enabled me to detach myself from variables that were beyond my control, such as the deaths of family members and travelling during the lockdown. This belief also reflected my submission to Allah in entrusting myself and my family's health in his hands. It provided me with a sense of relief that helped reduce my concern about the safety of my family members, in which I noticed an improvement in my mental well-being. In accordance with the narrative review, no study has investigated either the theme of faith or identity in maintaining personal resilience during COVID-19 to improve the mental well-being of students.

Spirituality During the Pandemic in the Narrative Review

The previous section analysed the influence of religious beliefs on protecting my mental health as an international student in the UK during the pandemic. To correlate this analysis with the findings of the narrative review, I focused on studies involving university students (home and international) in the UK, the USA and Canada. In this regard, the study of Aristeidou and Aristidou (2023) investigates the experiences of PhD students across various universities in the UK during the COVID-19 pandemic. Its primary objective is to identify factors contributing to mental health challenges among 1,780 PhD students. The study identified several coping strategies employed by PhD students to manage these challenges. Acceptance was the most widely reported strategy, with 84% of participants acknowledging the realities of their situation without denial. Seeking emotional support from peers, mentors or family members was another key strategy, helping to mitigate feelings of isolation and stress. Additionally, positive reframing – viewing negative experiences as opportunities for growth – was found to enhance resilience and coping capacity. Finally, mindfulness practices, such as prayer or meditation, were utilized by 73% of students, underscoring their effectiveness in managing stress and anxiety. These findings highlight the importance of adaptive coping mechanisms in supporting the mental well-being of PhD students during periods of significant disruption. Although Aristeidou and Aristidou (2023) reported that prayers and accepting reality were among the major strategies used by the students, they did not elaborate on their impact on improving mental well-being.

While the study by Aristeidou and Aristidou (2023) did not directly investigate the role of spirituality in building resilience among UK-based PhD students, their findings – particularly the emphasis on accepting reality and engaging in prayer – resonate with insights from the auto-hermeneutic approach. For instance, the role of faith in fostering resilience, such as embracing hardships as an act of submission to Allah and a demonstration of piety, exemplifies a form of reality acceptance influenced by the challenges of the COVID-19 pandemic. This alignment highlights the potential importance of spiritual practices in strengthening resilience during times of adversity.

Physical Exercise Strategy

The second strategy that helped tremendously to improve my mental health during the pandemic was physical fitness. I cycled for two hours a day from May 2020 to September 2020 and from April 2021 to September 2021. Cycling represented a stress-free activity because I was able to leave my house whilst the streets were empty. As described through my audio recording:

> Ah Alhamdulillah (thank God), at least I can sleep tonight after exhausting myself and emptying my mind through cycling. Thank God I was able to buy the bicycle before everything shut down.

This quotation demonstrates how cycling improved my sleeping patterns. My average sleeping time increased from two to three hours a day to an average of five hours. This positive correlation between cycling and my sleeping pattern became noticeable when I stopped for six months between the two periods (September 2020–April 2021) due to an increased percentage of COVID-19 cases and stricter lockdown regulations compared to the previously mentioned period (May 2020–September 2020).

The Effects of Physical Exercise on Improving Mental Well-Being

Within the narrative review, a few studies highlighted similar findings. Three studies addressing resilience and coping strategies were analysed (Al-Oraibi et al., 2022; Lai et al., 2020; Van Der Feltz-Cornelis et al., 2020). Varying strategies were reported in the findings of these studies: indoor exercises, reading, chatting with friends and family, cooking, video or mobile gaming, sports, spiritual support, listening to music and meditation. Lai et al. (2020) emphasized the importance of indoor exercises among international students because they helped them cope during self-isolation, and therefore, improved their psychological well-being and their studies. Similarly, Al-Oraibi et al. (2022) reported that indoor activities (e.g. watching movies, chatting with family and home physical exercises) assisted international students in the UK to cope with the stress of self-isolation. These indoor exercises, according to Al-Oraibi et al. (2022), were also perceived by the international students in the UK as distractions, which made the period of self-isolation appear shorter than it actually was. In line with Al-Oraibi et al. (2022) and Lai et al. (2020)'s findings on physical exercises and international students' resilience in the UK during the pandemic, the data gathered from my auto-hermeneutic approach also revealed that cycling maintained my resilience during the confinement periods.

The investigations conducted by Chen and Lucock (2022) as well as Saunders et al. (2022) similarly indicated that diminished physical activity resulting from lockdown measures significantly affected the psychological well-being of both international and home students. These results were corroborated in the cross-sectional research undertaken by Evans and colleagues (2021), which examined 297 doctoral students: the participants reported employing physical exercise as a strategy to mitigate their stress and anxiety, thereby enhancing their overall well-being during the COVID-19 pandemic. These findings are further reinforced by my personal documentation using the auto-hermeneutic approach. Cycling had a positive impact on my mental well-being by improving my sleep quality, which in turn alleviated my insomnia. Over time, I observed a noticeable improvement in my overall well-being compared to the period when my physical activity levels were significantly lower. This personal experience aligns with the broader evidence highlighting the critical role of physical activity in maintaining mental health, particularly during challenging times such as the COVID-19 pandemic.

The core experience illustrates the dynamic interaction between the individual and their environment. During the pandemic, two significant external stressors adversely affected my mental health: feelings of loneliness and the loss of family members due to COVID-19. These external factors contributed to a decline in my mental well-being, manifesting in symptoms such as increased depressive feelings and insomnia. To counteract these challenges and preserve psychological stability, I relied on internal motivators, including religious beliefs and physical fitness activities such as cycling. This interplay between external stressors and internal coping mechanisms reflects an interactive process shaped by my spatial context (being in the UK) and temporal context (during the pandemic). The integration of these elements served to stabilize my mental well-being (inner self) whenever it was threatened by external adversities.

Post-Experience

After the end of the third lockdown in July 2021 (Brown et al., 2021), the quarantine restrictions eased in the UK, which enabled me to travel to Algeria in July 2022. My trip allowed me to reflect on my experience as an international student in the UK after the pandemic. I reached the conclusion that loneliness and constant worry about family members during the pandemic were the two major psychological stressors affecting my mental well-being, which manifested in a prolonged state of insomnia for one year. Regarding the external stressors that solely emphasized the effects of the pandemic on my academic studies, I noticed a reduced level of stress after contacting five participants to proceed with my PhD project via a digital platform (Facebook). The post-experience findings are relatively shorter than the core-experience because my mental well-being improved significantly after the third lockdown, eliminating the need for audio recordings during this period.

Discussion

In line with the findings reported in this qualitative study (the auto-hermeneutic approach) and the studies selected for the narrative review, the commonalities reported across different studies reinforced the homogeneity between individuals despite different personal experiences. This led me to reflect on the concept of intersubjectivity in hermeneutics, which explains that knowledge is developed when investigating the influence of the surrounding environment on individual experiences (Smith et al., 2009). Intersubjectivity in this study appeared in the interplay between external factors (loneliness due to confinement, family loss due to the pandemic and change in the PhD project due to the closure of international borders), mental well-being (insomnia and stress) and the use of internal motivators to protect my psychological well-being when facing external adversities (religious beliefs and physical fitness exercises). The hegemony in intersubjectivity in this chapter was seen in the similar findings between my experience as an international student in the UK and the experiences of university students from the narrative review in the UK, the USA and Canada.

Findings from the auto-hermeneutic approach correlated with the results of the narrative review. From my personal experience as an international student pursuing a PhD in the UK during the pandemic, several psychological stressors were reported. First, academic uncertainty caused anxiety and mental distress. Particularly, the financial uncertainty associated with the expectation of finishing my PhD programme within a pre-determined timeline negatively affected my mental well-being. This finding aligns with the studies of Sverdlik et al. (2022), which spanned diverse geographical contexts (e.g. the USA, Canada, the UK, Australia, Asia and the Middle East), as well as the work of Aristeidou and Aristidou (2023) in the UK. Both studies identified financial concerns as a primary academic factor negatively impacting the mental health of international students.

The vital psychological stressors highlighted using an auto-hermeneutic approach reflected findings similar to Jackman et al. (2022). Among the challenges highlighted in their research, isolation, lack of motivation, reduced mental health and increased pressure were experienced by doctoral and early career researchers. Other factors such as loneliness, constant worry and insomnia also influenced mental health and well-being (Aristeidou & Aristidou, 2023; Jackman et al., 2022; Sverdlik et al., 2022). In this respect, studies selected for the narrative review reported similar findings to the auto-hermeneutic approach. For instance, both international and home students expressed anxiety, loneliness and mental distress (Al-Oraibi et al., 2022; Appleby et al., 2022; Burns et al., 2020; Catling et al., 2021; Chen & Lucock, 2022; Maleku et al., 2022; McGivern & Shepherd, 2022).

Data derived from both the auto-hermeneutic approach and narrative review consistently highlight that physical exercise significantly enhances students' mental well-being. This finding is further supported by studies on the general population (Wolf et al., 2021; Wood et al., 2022) and aligns with research conducted in Canada and the UK (Savage et al., 2020, 2021; Saunders et al., 2022), which emphasizes the positive impact of physical activity on university students' mental health. However, alternative coping strategies, such as video gaming, cooking or reading, were preferred by some students, as noted by Al-Oraibi et al. (2022) and Lai et al. (2020). Personally, incorporating cycling into my daily routine led to a marked improvement in my sleep patterns, which subsequently enhanced my mental well-being. My preference for cycling over other coping mechanisms was informed by scientific evidence demonstrating that physical exercise releases endorphins, which act as natural mood elevators, helping to alleviate stress and improve mental health during challenging periods.

Strengths, Limitations and Recommendations for Future Research

Like all research, this study has both strengths and limitations, with its contributions falling into two main categories: theoretical and methodological. Theoretically, this study underscores the value of adopting an interactionist approach to analyse the effects of external stressors on the psychological well-being of university students, as well as the role of internal motivators in fostering resilience and maintaining mental health stability during adversities. By applying the interactionist perspective to my experience as an international student in the UK, this research evaluated the extent to which external stressors impacted my mental well-being and how I utilized internal motivators to achieve psychological equilibrium amidst the challenges posed by the pandemic. This perspective enriches the existing literature on coping mechanisms during crises, particularly by introducing a novel theoretical contribution: the use of religious beliefs, specifically submission to Allah's will, as a strategy to counteract external stressors during the pandemic. Notably, the studies included in the narrative review did not address the role of faith among international students or its potential to enhance mental health during such unprecedented times.

Methodologically, the auto-hermeneutic approach proved highly effective in uncovering an under-researched dimension of religion as a coping mechanism during the pandemic. To the best of my knowledge, no research has employed this approach to explore the pandemic's impact on international students in the UK. This methodology provided a platform for my voice as an international Muslim student, representing a minority within a UK university, and allowed me to articulate how my faith played a pivotal role in sustaining my mental health during the pandemic. Furthermore, the auto-hermeneutic approach offers a humanistic dimension to data collection in health sciences, enabling individuals to freely express and reflect on their emotions and behaviours without the constraints of structured psychological tests. This method emphasizes qualitative depth and richness, as opposed to purely quantitative or clinical data, and facilitates reflective data collection through tools such as journals. By capturing rich (depth) and thick (length) data, the auto-hermeneutic approach allows professionals to analyse first-hand experiences without influencing participants' responses, as is often the case in structured or semi-structured interviews. This methodological contribution accentuates the potential of auto-hermeneutics to provide nuanced insights into the psychological and emotional dimensions of health and well-being.

Limitations

As outlined in the methods section, my emotions and thoughts were recorded on four separate occasions, driven by the need to articulate my concerns during the pandemic. This approach ensured the credibility of the data analysed in the core-experience section, as it was documented through voice recordings. In contrast, the findings in the post-experience section relied solely on recollection, which may have compromised their depth and accuracy. This discrepancy is evident in the inconsistency between the two subsections: the core experience contains rich, detailed data, while the post-experience is comparatively brief and less comprehensive. This inconsistency represents a limitation of the study. To address this issue in future research employing the auto-hermeneutic approach, it is recommended that data – whether oral or written – be consistently recorded throughout both core and post-experience phases to ensure the credibility and quality of the findings.

Another potential limitation of this study lies in its sampling, as it explores the impact of the pandemic from the perspective of a single international PhD student in the UK using an auto-hermeneutic approach. However, it is important to note that single case studies are a recognized and credible methodological approach, particularly in the field of health sciences. Such studies can provide valuable insights and broaden the theoretical and methodological scope of research, offering a detailed and nuanced understanding of individual experiences that may inform broader applications. Thus, while the sample size may appear limited, the depth and rigor of the auto-hermeneutic approach lend credibility to the findings and contribute meaningfully to the existing literature.

Recommendations

The current research did not aim to compare the experiences of international students across different countries (e.g. the UK, the USA and Canada) or examine the influence of these specific contexts on both international and domestic students simultaneously. As such, future research could explore the correlation between geographical locations and the experiences of university students, considering both international and home student populations. Additionally, while existing studies have predominantly focused on the academic achievement and mental well-being of students during the pandemic, there is a notable gap in research addressing the financial challenges they faced. Future studies could therefore investigate the impact of socioeconomic status, particularly among international students, on their mental well-being during crises. Finally, further research could delve into the role of faith in fostering resilience during periods of stress and adversity, an area that remains underexplored in the current literature. These directions would provide a more comprehensive understanding of the multifaceted challenges faced by students during global crises and inform targeted support strategies.

Conclusion

This study enhances the understanding of the COVID-19 pandemic's impact on one student's mental health well-being by employing auto-hermeneutics and a narrative review to gather and analyse data. Key findings identified several psychological stressors affecting university students, including loneliness, concerns about family members, a loss of direction, academic uncertainty, reduced physical activity and socioeconomic challenges. By focusing on the self (personal experience), this research introduces novel insights to the field of health sciences. Unlike many existing studies that treat international students in the UK, Canada and the USA as a homogeneous group, this study highlights the individual experiences of a single international student, shedding light on unique challenges such as financial pressures and time constraints faced by sponsored students. Additionally, it underscores the role of physical fitness as a widely adopted coping strategy during the pandemic, benefiting both international and domestic students. Importantly, the auto-hermeneutic approach revealed that religious beliefs also functioned as a resilience strategy, an area that warrants further exploration. Future research could investigate the conceptual relationship between religiosity and mental well-being, as this remains an under-researched topic. Overall, this study demonstrates that, despite individual and regional differences, international and domestic students shared common mental health challenges during the pandemic, emphasizing the universality of their experiences.

References

Adams, T. E., & Manning, J. (2015). Autoethnography and family research. *Journal of Family Theory &Amp; Review*, 7(4), 350–366. https://doi.org/10.1111/jftr.12116.

Al-Oraibi, A., Fothergill, L., Yildirim, M., Knight, H., Carlisle, S., O'Connor, M., Briggs, L., Morling, J., Corner, J., Ball, J. K., Denning, C., Vedhara, K., & Blake, H. (2022).

Exploring the psychological impacts of COVID-19 social restrictions on international university students: A qualitative study. *International Journal of Environmental Research and Public Health, 19*(13), 1–19. https://doi.org/10.3390/ijerph1913763.

Appleby, J. A., King, N., Saunders, K. E., Bast, A., Rivera, D., Byun, J., Cunningham, S., Khera, C., & Duffy, A. C. (2022). Impact of the COVID-19 pandemic on the experience and mental health of university students studying in Canada and the UK: A cross-sectional study. *BMJ Open, 12*(1), Article e050187. https://doi.org/10.1136/bmjopen-2021-050187.

Aristeidou, M., & Aristidou, A. (2023). Research disruption during PhD studies and its impact on mental health: Implications for research and university policy. *PLoS ONE, 18*(10), e0291555. https://doi.org/10.1371/journal.pone.0291555.

Burns, D., Dagnall, N., & Holt, M. (2020). Assessing the impact of the COVID-19 pandemic on student wellbeing at universities in the United Kingdom: A conceptual analysis. *Frontiers in Education, 5*, 1–10. https://doi.org/10.3389/feduc.2020.582882.

Carù, A., & Cova, B. (2015). Co-creating the collective service experience. *Journal of Service Management, 26*(2), 276–294. https://doi.org/10.1108/JOSM-07-2014-0170

Catling, J. C., Bayley, A., Begum, Z., Wardzinski, C., & Wood, A. (2022). Effects of the COVID-19 lockdown on mental health in a UK student sample. *BMC Psychology, 10*(1), 1–7. https://doi.org/10.1186/s40359-022-00732-9.

Chen T., & Lucock M. (2022). The mental health of university students during the COVID-19 pandemic: An online survey in the UK. *PLoS ONE, 17*(1), 1–17.

Ellway, B. P. W., & Dean, A. M. (2016). The reciprocal intertwining of practice and experience in value creation. *Marketing Theory, 16*(3), 299–324. https://doi.org/10.1177/1470593116636088.

Evans, K. E., Holmes, M. R., Prince, D. M., & Groza, V. (2021). Social work doctoral student well-being during the COVID-19 pandemic: A descriptive study. *International Journal of Doctoral Studies, 16*, 569–592. https://doi.org/10.28945/4840.

Evans, S., Alkan, E., Bhangoo, J. K., Tenenbaum, H., & Ng-Knight, T. (2021). Effects of the COVID-19 lockdown on mental health, wellbeing, sleep, and alcohol use in a UK student sample. *Psychiatry Research, 298*, 1–7. https://doi.org/10.1016/j.psychres.2021.113819.

Galderisi, S., Heinz, A., Kastrup, M., Beezhold, J., & Sartorius, N. (2015). Toward a new definition of mental health. *World Psychiatry, 14*(2), 231–233. https://doi.org/10.1002/wps.20231

Gorichanaz, T. (2017). Auto-hermeneutics: A phenomenological approach to information experience. *Library & Information Science Research, 39*(1), 1–7. https://doi.org/10.1016/j.lisr.2017.01.001.

Grant, M. J., & Booth, A. (2009). A typology of reviews: An analysis of 14 review types and associated methodologies. *Health Information & Libraries Journal, 26*(2), 91–108. https://doi.org/10.1111/j.1471-1842.2009.00848.x

Green, B. N., Johnson, C. D., & Adams, A. (2006). Writing narrative literature reviews for peer-reviewed journals: Secrets of the trade. *Journal of Chiropractic Medicine, 5*(3), 101–117. https://doi.org/10.1016/S0899-3467(07)60142-6

Jackman, P. C., Sanderson, R., Haughey, T. J., Brett, C. E., White, N., Zile, A., & Byrom, N. C. (2022). The impact of the first COVID-19 lockdown in the UK for doctoral and early career researchers. *Higher Education*, *84*(4), 705–722. https://doi.org/10.1007/s10734-021-00795-4.

Lai, A. Y., Lee, L., Wang, M. P., Feng, Y., Lai, T. T., Ho, L. M., Lam, V. S., Ip, M. S., & Lam, T. H. (2020). Mental health impacts of the COVID-19 pandemic on international university students, related stressors, and coping strategies. *Frontiers in Psychiatry*, *11*, 1–13. https://doi.org/10.3389/fpsyt.2020.584240.

Maleku, A., Kim, Y. K., Kirsch, J., Um, M. Y., Haran, H., Yu, M., & Moon, S. S. (2022). The hidden minority: Discrimination and mental health among international students in the US during the COVID-19 pandemic. *Health & Social Care in the Community*, *30*(5). https://doi.org/10.1111/hsc.13683.

McGivern, P., & Shepherd, J. (2022). The impact of COVID-19 on UK university students: Understanding the interconnection of issues experienced during lockdown. *Power and Education*, *14*(3), 218–227. https://doi.org/10.1177/17577438221104227.

Méndez-López, M. (2013). Autoethnography as a research method: Advantages, limitations and criticisms. *Colombian Applied Linguistics Journal*, *15*, 279–287. https://doi.org/10.14483/udistrital.jour.calj.2013.2.a09.

Office for National Statistics (2020). Coronavirus and the impact on students in higher education in England: September to December 2020. https://www.ons.gov.uk/peoplepopulationandcommunity/educationandchildcare/articles/coronavirusandtheimpactonstudentsinhighereducationinenglandseptembertodecember2020/2020-12-21

Pyhältö, K., Tikkanen, L., & Anttila, H. (2023). The influence of the COVID-19 pandemic on PhD candidates' study progress and study wellbeing. *Higher Education Research & Development*, *42*(2), 413–426. https://doi.org/10.1080/07294360.2022.2063816.

Roth, T. (2007). Insomnia: Definition, prevalence, etiology, and consequences. *Journal of Clinical Sleep Medicine*, *3*(5), 7–10. https://www.ncbi.nlm.nih.gov/pmc/articles/PMC1978319/pdf/jcsm.3.5.s7.pdf.

Savage, M. J., Hennis, P. J., Magistro, D., Donaldson, J., Healy, L. C., & James, R. M. (2021). Nine months into the COVID-19 pandemic: A longitudinal study showing mental health and movement behaviours are impaired in UK students. *International Journal of Environmental Research and Public Health*, *18*(6). https://doi.org/10.3390/ijerph18062930

Savage, M. J., James, R., Magistro, D., Donaldson, J., Healy, L. C., Nevill, M., & Hennis, P. J. (2020). Mental health and movement behaviour during the COVID-19 pandemic in UK university students: Prospective cohort study. *Mental Health and Physical Activity*, *19*, 1–6. https://doi.org/10.1016/j.mhpa.2020.100357.

Smith, J. A., Flowers, P., & Larkin, M. (2009). *Interpretative Phenomenological Analysis: Theory, Method and Research.* Sage Publications.

Smith, J. A., & Nizza, I. E. (2022). *Essentials of interpretative phenomenological analysis.* American Psychological Association.

Sverdlik, A., Hall, N. C., & Vallerand, R. J. (2022). Doctoral students and COVID-19: Exploring challenges, academic progress, and well-being. *Educational Psychology*, *43*(5), 545–560. https://doi.org/10.1080/01443410.2022.2091749

UK Parliament POST (21 July 2021). *Mental Health Impacts of the COVID-19 Pandemic on Adults*. https://post.parliament.uk/research-briefings/post-pn-0648/.

Van der Feltz-Cornelis, C. M., Varley, D., Allgar, V. L., & De Beurs, E. (2020). Workplace stress, presenteeism, absenteeism, and resilience amongst university staff and students in the COVID-19 lockdown. *Frontiers in Psychiatry, 11*. https://doi.org/10.3389/fpsyt.2020.588803.

Wall, S. (2008). Easier said than done: Writing an autoethnography. *International Journal of Qualitative Methods, 7*(1), 38–53. https://doi.org/10.1177/160940690800700103.

Wolf, S., Seiffer, B., Zeibig, J. M., Welkerling, J., Brokmeier, L., Atrott, B., Ehring, T., & Schuch, F. B. (2021). Is physical activity associated with less depression and anxiety during the COVID-19 pandemic? A rapid systematic review. *Sports Medicine, 51*(8), 1771–1783. https://www.ncbi.nlm.nih.gov/pmc/articles/PMC8060908/.

Wood, C. J., Barton, J., & Smyth, N. (2022). A cross-sectional study of physical activity behaviour and associations with wellbeing during the UK coronavirus lockdown. *Journal of Health Psychology, 27*(6), 1432–1444. https://www.ncbi.nlm.nih.gov/pmc/articles/PMC9036158/.

World Health Organization (WHO, 2026). *Mental health*. https://www.who.int/health-topics/mental-health#tab=tab_1

Zavlis, O., Butter, S., Bennett, K., Hartman, T. K., Hyland, P., Mason, L., McBride, O., Murphy, J., Gibson-Miller, J., Levita, L., Martinez, A. P., Shevlin, M., Stocks, T. V. A., Vallières, F., & Bentall, R. P. (2021). How does the COVID-19 pandemic impact on population mental health? A network analysis of COVID influences on depression, anxiety and traumatic stress in the UK population. *Psychological Medicine, 52*(16), 3825–3833. https://doi.org/10.1017/S0033291721000635.

Zhou, M., & Kan, M. Y. (2021). The varying impacts of COVID-19 and its related measures in the UK: A year in review. *PLOS ONE, 16*(9), 1–21. https://doi.org/10.1371/journal.pone.0257286.

· 4 ·

THE NEED TO RECONSIDER THE OCCUPATIONAL RIGHTS OF LOW-WAGE ESSENTIAL WORKERS POST-PANDEMIC

Steven Kupidy and Lynn Shaw

The important role essential workers play in achieving both public health and economic interests was underscored during the COVID-19 pandemic. The representation of who is identified as an essential worker by the public and decision makers unexpectedly expanded from front-line healthcare and first responders to include low-wage workers who were unaccustomed to this role. This study utilized critical discourse analysis methodology to examine the discursive practices used in Canadian newspaper articles within three distinct time periods during the COVID-19 pandemic, ranging from March 2020 up to and including January 2021. The study revealed implications and challenges to the underlying purposes of well-being, belonging and continually developing in paid work occupations when work identities shifted from non-essential to essential for low-wage workers. The complex and shifting identity of the essential worker during the pandemic challenged historical understandings, that is, definitions and social valuations of essential workers, through the response to the COVID-19 pandemic. Findings further elucidated the need to address unanticipated injustices through the consideration of occupational rights for all workers identified as essential during a global and/or national crisis. Future consideration of an expanded definition is required for essential work to encompass both work and workers. An expanded definition will assist in guiding decision makers on how best to utilize and support essential workers in Canadian society before, during and after a crisis by highlighting the inclusion of occupational rights as a framework to reduce any undue hardships or restrictions these essential workers may experience. In particular, the findings raise important opportunities for employers, unions, worker advocates and governments to re-examine policies, hiring practices and education to promote worker identity shifts, occupational worker rights and to sustain health and safety.

The COVID-19 pandemic impacted workers around the world. In response to COVID-19, one of the significant shifts affecting workers was the way work was valued by governments and society. From the governmental perspective in Canada, the federal public health agency, in collaboration with provincial health authorities, limited physical access to sectors of the economy and areas within communities to prevent viral spread within the population. Public health orders identified principles such as the maintenance of specific services essential to respond to the pandemic, for example, protective services and urgent care services (Public Safety Canada, 2021). However, the enforcement of border closures, stay-at-home and quarantine initiatives and the closure of businesses deemed non-essential (Canadian Public Health Association, 2021) impacted employable Canadians' ability to work freely and safely. Specifically, the jobs and industries identified as essential by federal and provincial governments were balanced against ensuring access to resources and services to maintain public health and safety (Public Safety Canada, 2021). This shift included a large group of low-wage workers, now considered essential, which was previously seen as non-essential outside the context of the COVID-19 pandemic. Further, the shift and disruptions experienced by those newly identified low-wage essential workers during the COVID-19 pandemic contributed to a change in the expression of occupational rights of low-wage essential workers. Hammell (2008) defined occupational rights " the right of all people to engage in meaningful occupations that contribute positively to their own well-being and the well-being of their communities." (p. 61).

This chapter[1] aims to provide additional context surrounding the essential worker by historically examining the rationale for essential work within society and how essential workers were represented in previous pandemics up to and including the COVID-19 pandemic. In addition, the shaping role media plays in the development and support of social issues is presented as a backdrop informing this discursive inquiry into the social issue of low-wage workers as essential workers and the impact on occupational rights.

Background on Essential Worker Classification in Canada

The primary tenets for the development of workers' rights and the need to classify some workers as essential were initially established through the labour movement advocated at the end of World War I (International Labour Organization, 2023).

1 This chapter is based on Steven Kupidy's (2022) Masters of Science thesis.

The labour movement and workers' rights expanded through the creation of the International Labour Organization (ILO) outlined in the Treaty of Versailles in 1919, where "the belief that universal and lasting peace can be accomplished only if it is based on social justice" (ILO, 2023, para 3). Decent work was seen as a cornerstone to lasting peace in the post-war society of the founding country members. Although Canada did not participate in the initial draft of the ILO constitution, Canada was a founding member, joining the ILO in 1919 (ILO, 2023). Canada was also a temporary headquarters for the ILO from 1940–1948, being housed at McGill University in Montreal, Quebec, which reflected the country's deep support and involvement with the ILO (2023). The ILO treaty and subsequent documents further developed and delineated that some workers are considered more critical to the maintenance of safety and security of society compared to other workers and need to be identified as essential (Pankart, 1980, as cited in Muñoz, 2014). To assist workers, employers and governments in the economic and social identification of essential worker groups, the ILO proposed an initial list of work that may be considered essential, including hospital services, electrical services, water supply services, telephone services, police and armed forces, firefighting services, public or private prison services, food provision to school age pupils', school cleaning and air traffic control (ILO, 2006). The identification of essential worker groups remained largely unchanged by evolving world contexts for the twentieth century, reinforcing roles and identities that have become familiar in society, representing essential work such as nurses, doctors, law enforcement, firefighters and workers supporting critical infrastructure. Low-wage workers, for example, grocery store clerks, warehouse workers and childcare workers, did not see their roles added to the list of essential labour prior to COVID-19.

In early 2020, the emergence of COVID-19 in Canada challenged federal and regional governments to act to protect the safety and security of its citizens. Expanding the number of workers considered essential workers to maintain access to certain resources and services was an unfamiliar governmental approach not seen in previous pandemic responses. The Government of Canada's response to COVID-19 resulted in the maintenance of the previously outlined critical sectors developed by the Canadian government (Government of Canada, 2015). However, an expanded group emerged under each sector which included workers such as grocery store clerks, truck transportation drivers, plumbers, construction workers, warehouse workers and childcare for essential workers (Canadian Human Rights Commission, 2021). These newly identified essential worker groups were classified due to the government's responses to COVID-19 and not willfully via the occupational choice of workers, as highlighted by Parks et al. (2020).

One of the core ideas used in designating a service essential implies that withholding that service would result in an imminent threat to the health and safety of communities (Muñoz, 2014), which is a consequence most newly classified essential workers did not knowingly acknowledge at the outset of employment pre-COVID-19 (Parks et al., 2020). This expanded classification complicated these newly anointed essential workers' ability to safely perform their work while assuming additional personal and economic risks. For example, Parks et al. (2020) highlighted that most food system workers did not knowingly sign up to be working on the front lines of a pandemic where they found themselves often ill-prepared with adequate knowledge and appropriate levels of personal protective equipment (PPE) to protect their health and well-being beyond typical workplace expectations. Whereas other workers deemed to be essential prior to the pandemic made choices to join law enforcement or become firefighters, nurses or doctors where health risks are explicit, these *new* essential workers did not.

Pandemics and the Literature on Essential Workers

In past pandemics, for example, severe Acute Respiratory 344 Syndrome (SARS) in 2003 and H1N1 (bird flu) in 2009, there has been research surrounding the impact on front line healthcare workers as an identified essential worker group (Institute of Labour Economics, 2020) and their response to the pandemic (Bai et al., 2004; Matsuishi et al., 2012; Wong et al., 2012). Gershon et al. (2010) expanded the essential worker group to include not only hospital workers but police department personnel, emergency medical service personnel, fire department personnel, public health department workers and prison officers. This study was unique in that it offered an examination pertaining to a larger group of essential workers where previously referenced studies limited their study populations to health care only. It was limited in scope focusing only on factors affecting the willingness of these essential workers to report for duty during the SARS pandemic and did not focus on the health and well-being or injustices faced by essential workers (Gershon et al., 2010). Low-wage workers, for example, taxi drivers or grocery store clerks that had been identified as essential during the COVID-19 pandemic were absent as a research population from the literature search conducted pertaining to previous pandemic responses.

In the context of the COVID-19 pandemic, new groups of essential workers emerged that included food system workers (Parks et al., 2020), postal delivery, construction, taxi drivers, long haul truck drivers (Benhamou & Piedra, 2020), community home health support workers and homeless/shelter workers (Williams et al., 2020). These workers were identified in the literature and in the news media as essential workers in the COVID-19 pandemic response, and in

Quebec, the government referred to these frontline workers as "guardian angels".[2] Parks et al. (2020) posited that the pandemic created a situation where low-wage or low-skilled workers not traditionally identified as essential workers (outside the context of a pandemic) may have experienced injustices and hardships such as increased anxiety around workplace safety, a lack of appropriate PPE, and little to no sick pay or sick days. For example, Benhamou and Piedra (2020) highlighted that access to union representation, knowledge surrounding health risks and access to PPE could not be guaranteed during COVID-19 for low-wage workers.

Media Discourse and the Shaping of Public Importance on Social Issues

The choice of inquiry using the news media, for example, newspapers, radio, television and news websites, can have several effects on readers. These effects contributed to the shift in classifying low-wage workers as essential workers. For instance, the effect of informing, agenda-setting, framing and persuading (Collins et al., 2006) can lead readers to think differently about what social issue is important in society, including who is seen as essential and non-essential. News media informs by providing orientation surrounding issues and events to the readership. Media can agenda-set and this effect is described as one of the most noted features of news media (Collins et al., 2006). Agenda setting is defined as the "media's ability to raise the salience of novel or existing issues, and the corresponding level of importance the public assigns to these issues" (Cohen, 1963; McCombs & Shaw, 1972; Otten, 1992 as cited in Collins et al., 2006, p. 90). For instance, this effect works when the media raises awareness of issues and then the public assigns importance to the issues, such as the valuing of the work of non-essential workers. Furthermore, the media engages in agenda-setting by stressing and framing certain aspects of the story to underpin the importance of that issue. The media, through these processes, can persuade public perception and understanding of the importance of the issues they are presenting (Collins et al., 2006). News media can extend these described power domains through various discursive strategies utilized in written texts.

---

2 This rhetoric of referring to essential workers as "guardian angels" was a psychological play to encourage individuals to participate in "the greater good" and morally employ individuals to participate in something outside of themselves. Quite simply, it was a form of manipulation – as further evidenced by the Quebec Government's decision to prevent asylum seekers working as essential workers in the province from accessing the Canadian Government's permanent residence programme (Rafiquddin, 2021; Schué, 2025).

The authors of this chapter posited that the shaping of the essential worker discourse during the COVID-19 pandemic was framed and influenced through discursive practices, that is, communication and language styles. Assumptions, representations, intertextuality and labelling represent some examples of communication and language styles commonly used to construct and convey an intended meaning found in Canadian news media written texts. This framing resulted in the politicization of the essential worker by the news media. Politicization is defined by Kari et al. (2019, p. 273) as "a social process through which the way how certain issues are governed by political institutions is contested". Being identified as an essential worker and critical to preserving the life and health of communities during the COVID-19 pandemic may have introduced factors influencing the change, disruption and maintenance of occupational rights for some newly classified essential workers.

It is through a focus on occupational rights that potential inequities and injustices, like the social injustices, for example, unsafe and inhumane working environments and a lack of workplace benefits and supports, can be highlighted and addressed (Hammell & Beagan, 2017). The lack of consideration to occupational rights (right of choice, right to work) added increased risk to personal health and reduced autonomy in paid work occupations for low-wage workers as the essentiality of their work required some to assume unsafe working conditions. Thus, this research investigated the shaping of low-wage workers as essential workers during the COVID-19 pandemic that were framed in the news media texts as a method to highlight these injustices experienced by low-wage workers during the COVID-19 pandemic.

Methodology in Critical Discourse Research

The purpose of this research is to critically examine the news media's discursive practices utilized during the early months of the COVID-19 pandemic related to the identity of the essential worker. The examination of the written texts surrounding essential workers during the COVID-19 pandemic used critical discourse analysis (CDA), informed primarily by critical discourse methodologies of Gee (2005), Fairclough (2003) and Wodak (2001). These authors have been recognized for their contributions surrounding critical discourse methodology. CDA, in its simplest form, is a study of language (Gee, 2005). Discourse analysis can be applied to a variety of different written forms, such as newspapers, advertising and magazine articles. Discursive practices are used by writers to reflect ideologies or social constructions in the analysis of texts considers (Gee, 2005), for example, intertextuality, nomination, social languages, assumptions and representations. These practices are then used in discourse analysis of text to understand the meaning and intentions and how they shape new understandings.

Intertextuality refers to one spoken or written text being directly used or alluded to in another spoken or written text, and it also considers both the writer and the reader in making meaning of the text (Gee, 2005). Referential/Nomination refers to the use of linguistic devices including membership categorization (Bakker, 1997; Sacks, 1992; as cited in Wodak & Meyer, 2001), metaphors and metonymies and synecdoche (figures of speech). Labelling is also a linguistic practice used to describe a person or group, in particular, highlighting positive or negative traits (Wing-Chun Ng, 2020). Social languages, according to Gee (2005, p. 35), are shaped through different varieties of language, in a text, the speaker or writer demonstrates differing identities that contribute to shaping different meanings. Assumptions refer to the implicitness that accompanies written texts or what is the meaning behind the text used (Gee, 2005). Representations refer to elements of a social event that are either included or excluded and which elements are given the most prominence in the text (Fairclough, 2003).

Pertaining to this research, written news media articles from March 2020 to January 2021 were used to examine the construction of the new essential worker. There were two questions that informed this research:

1) What discursive strategies were utilized by the Canadian news media through written texts that contributed to the discourse surrounding essential workers, including low-wage, low-skilled workers, during the early phases of the COVID-19 pandemic?
2) What was the impact, if any, on the attainment and/or maintenance of occupational rights for low-wage, low-skilled essential workers during the early months of the COVID-19 pandemic in Canada?

Data Selection and Inclusion/Exclusion Strategies

Factiva, an international news database, was used in this study, given its comprehensiveness as a source of written newspaper articles globally. Using the Factiva database, a keyword search using the words pandemic, essential workers, frontline workers, COVID-19 was conducted within three defined time periods with a focus on Canadian newsprint: period one (1 March–30 April 2020), period two (1 May–31 July 2020) and period three (1 November–31 January 2021). The rationale for establishing three periods was to examine any shifts or transformations surrounding the essential worker discourse between time periods. These periods also represent distinct shifts in the federal and provincial governments' response to managing the pandemic. The time period of August to October 2020 was indistinguishable from period 2 regarding federal and provincial policy proclamations and thus not specifically examined.

The inclusion criteria for document selection were: (1) a major daily newspaper, (2) an English publication and (3) top ten distribution numbers in Canada. English-speaking major daily newspapers represent most of the daily circulated newsprint in Canada (News Media Canada, 2020) and are the broadest source of newspaper articles to sample for this research project. The top ten English-speaking newspapers in Canada based on circulation numbers were initially identified as primary document sources. However, the largest publications based on circulation numbers for Quebec (English speaking), Eastern Canada and the Northern territories were added, and three publications were removed (due to regional duplication) to capture a broader geographical representation.

Based on the initial inclusion criteria, eighty-seven articles were identified. The researchers further applied exclusion criteria in a phased article selection process and reduced the number to sixty-three in phase 2 and eventually down to six per time period at phase 3 (Tables 4.1–4.4). The remaining six articles from each period were hand-selected by the researcher. Value based judgements surrounding the process of text selection are permitted in CDA (Wodak & Meyer, 2001). The primary criteria for the hand selected articles included: (1) the inclusion of articles in geographies that may have been underrepresented in the first two exclusion phases, (2) a diversity in the writers representing both employed and freelance writers with diverse educational and professional backgrounds, (3) a balance of news article and opinion formatted articles and (4) articles that reflected a special interest of the researchers related to public policy.

Table 4.1: Phased Application of Exclusion Criteria

Phase 1	Phase 2	Phase 3
Classified as newswire or staff wire (summary story) Essential workers not highlighted in COVID-19 Duplicate article with a different title	The identification of frontline or essential workers was not the subject of the article, but mentioned incidentally (not the focus of the story)	Six articles hand selected by the researchers

Table 4.2: News Articles Selected from 1 March to 30 April 2020 (Period 1)

Author	News Title	Publication
Monesbraaten, L.	COVID-19 policies create child-care crunch for essential workers	Toronto Star
Lysack, A.; White, M.	Even as their role in fighting COVID-19 has become clear, childcare workers remain an afterthought	Toronto Star
Boyle, J.; Pagliaro, T.	First homeless shelter workers tested positive for COVID-19, sparking calls for increased protection.	Toronto Star
Benzie, R.	Ontario to increase inspections at construction sites and grocery stores to ensure workers are safe.	Toronto Star
Saltman, J.	Planned cuts would hurt essential workers; Advocates urge other Translink options.	Vancouver Province
Johnson, L.	Province expands child-care eligibility to include all workers deemed essential.	Edmonton Journal

Table 4.3: News Articles Selected from 1 May to 31 July 2020 (Period 2)

Author	News Title	Publication
Tumilty, R.	Are you essential? In Canada, it depends where one lives; Federal top-up pay.	National Post
Speer, S.	Never forget the dignity of our essential workers.	National Post
Ryan, D.	New schools getting the "essentials" right; Classrooms for children of front-line workers paving the way to a supportive, team-oriented future.	Vancouver Province
Winnipeg Free Press Editorial Board	No serenade, but wage hike is warranted.	Winnipeg Free Press
Keller, J.	Parents weigh options as Alberta daycares prepare to reopen as early as May 14.	Globe and Mail
Lett, D.	Risk payment plan sure to exclude worthy workers.	Winnipeg Free Press

Table 4.4: News Articles Selected from 1 November to 31 January 2021 (Period 3)

Author	News Title	Publication
Sellar, C.	A taxing pandemic for taxi drivers.	Winnipeg Free Press
Kennedy, B.	City looks to provide emergency child-care to essential workers during post-holiday remote learning.	Toronto Star
Dewhirst, T.	Essential businesses are a blurred and contested concept.	Toronto Star
Brar, A. Dr., Daniel, M., Dr., Sra, G.	"I am scared to take a day off whether sick or not." The voiceless warehouse workers in Peel and how COVID-19 has silenced them even more.	Toronto Star
Brar, A. Dr.	Ontario continues to refuse legislation for paid sick days, says CRSB is enough. But that option is inaccessible for many. Here's the difference.	Toronto Star
Vohra-Miller, S, Dosani, N. Dr., Marwaha, S. Dr., Bulle, S.	Ontario locks down on Boxing Day, but essential workers still work. Without protections like paid sick leave, it just won't work.	Toronto Star

Data Analysis

The discourse analysis of each news article was conducted over multiple readings and was informed by the methods and data analysis processes established by Gee (2005), Fairclough (2003) and Wodak (2001). The purpose of the initial readings was to reveal predominant discursive tools that were used within these written texts, and they were identified as assumptions, representations, intertextuality and labelling. In this step, evidence of their use was highlighted in each text. The next step was to make sense of what were the most prominent discourse(s) shaped in each time period. The final step of analysis was to consider common themes or shifts in the representation of low-wage workers across all three time periods.

Findings

The texts analysed over the three time periods from March 2020 to January 2021 resulted in two primary themes emerging. Firstly, the politicization of the essential worker during COVID-19 is discussed by various writers. Secondly, over the time periods, the identity of the essential workers was constructed to include low-wage and low-skilled workers. Both influenced the essential worker discourse during the COVID-19 pandemic.

The Re-construction of the Essential Worker Identity

Early in the analysis of period one articles, a strong representation of the essential and dominant nature of healthcare was established through prominence in the texts. Healthcare is referenced as an essential service in 100% of period one articles, 80% of period 2 articles, and 30% of period three articles. This discursive representation was reinforced through intertextuality. Gee (2005) defines intertextuality as spoken or written text being directly used or alluded to in another spoken or written text. Intertextuality was noted through the direct and indirect reporting of information, and through the researcher noting the absence of other non-healthcare essential worker groups in the texts. This revealed the predominance of the strong representation surrounding essential healthcare workers, for example, nurses, as being highly valued and critically important to society, especially as the pandemic started.

As the articles progressed through the time periods, the discursive use of nomination by the writers expanded to include the positive traits of both healthcare workers and some non-healthcare workers collectively. Efforts were made to increase the societal value of low-wage workers through association with established, valued healthcare workers. For instance, this was done through statements such as "overwhelming public expressions of admiration and respect for those workers who have manned our front lines of our hospitals, sustained our food supply, delivered our packages" (Speer, 2020, para. 3). In this textual example, the writer establishes the predominance and importance of the front-line hospital workers by placing this group first in the list. There were discursive attempts by several writers, albeit not collectively, to establish some sense of a homogeneous collective representation or broadened membership categorization of the essential worker. Through the news media, the establishment of a collective identity and a sense of belonging to this essential worker category for the low-wage worker appears to be a critical bridge from a societal value perspective. These discursive practices helped connect what was historically identified as an essential worker, for example, nurses and first responders, with the other essential workers required during the COVID-19 response, for example, grocery store clerks, warehouse workers and community workers.

Establishment of a Sense of Belonging within the Low-Wage Essential Worker Identity

Parks et al. (2020) noted that the sense of belonging or social acceptance typically eluded low-wage, low-skilled workers, including grocery store clerks, food service workers and warehouse workers. The authors (Parks et al., 2020) did not speculate as to what may have contributed to this observation. This lack of belonging may be a result of their perceived lack of association with other more notable essential worker groups. For instance, several writers highlighted low-wage workers as humble or apprehensive of attention. Several writers utilized the discursive practice of nomination, that of highlighting specific traits of low-wage workers including, "they're unaccustomed to accolades for their efforts" (Winnipeg Free Press Editorial Board, 2020, para. 9) and "It's our duty. We are also front-liners" (Sellar, 2020, para. 12). These two textual examples, through intertextual phrases (direct and indirect reporting), categorize low-wage workers as being both self-effacing and self-sacrificial. This self-effacement continued to be reinforced discursively through labelling as writers emphasized that many worked shifts that did not end with an orchestra, serenades or the banging of pots to show support, contrary to public displays for healthcare workers (Sellar, 2020). Establishing a sense of camaraderie through a shared identity for the reader, for example, nurses and grocery clerks sharing a common essential role, also results in the reader assuming a form of equality within the essential worker group. Being seen as important as nurses and other front-line healthcare workers may have been part of the intrinsic justification required for low-wage essential workers to continue to show up for work during the pandemic, despite facing a disproportionate level of health risk along with lower wages. Discursively engraining this value assumption of belonging by association motivated low-wage essential workers living within their concomitant socioeconomic realities to remain working.

> What has been interesting though is our definition of essentiality in a crisis has differed greatly from how society normally thinks about it. So-called low skilled jobs like grocery clerks, janitors, and gas station attendants have been elevated to essential and various high skilled workers have been relegated to work-from-home status or shut down entirely. (Speer, 2020, para. 2)

Speer (2020) discursively establishes the existential assumption that being seen as essential is conditional. Based on this, the authors of this paper posit that if the right conditions are met, any worker could be elevated to essential at any given time. Thus, the conditions for low-wage workers to be seen as essential are some form of crisis. Because of the COVID-19 crisis, these low-wage workers faced "a level of risk that was never inherent in their job descriptions" (Lett, 2020, para. 9).

It is outside the scope of this research project to infer whether any of these low-wage workers viewed themselves as essential prior to the COVID-19 pandemic. However, one writer provides some insight as to how society implicitly determines the value of work, noting that "the modern economy pays significant financial returns for certain aptitudes, credentials, and skills" (Speer, 2020, para. 5). Additionally, Speer (2020) describes that "it reflects an unhealthy tendency in modern society to value people based on their income and status" (para. 6). Given these statements, it is important to consider that even if some of these low-wage workers identified themselves as essential, this perspective was not likely reflected through any form of societal acknowledgement prior to the pandemic.

Also, the assumption that the COVID-19 pandemic introduced a health risk to low-wage workers that was not present prior to the pandemic is reinforced by writers and politicians. "If you're risking your health to keep this country moving and you're making minimum wage, you deserve a raise" (Tumilty, 2020, para. 1) was proclaimed by Prime Minister, Justin Trudeau. This portrayal fails to acknowledge that making minimum wage is a social determinant of health on its own and working for minimum wage is itself a health risk factor as this adds financial challenges to meeting one's basic needs for example, adequate food and housing. The lack of recognition that low-wage workers are deserving of a raise downplays the concomitant socioeconomic risks faced by low-wage workers. Several writers emphasized what existed, as far as working conditions, prior to COVID-19 by highlighting that, "minimum wage in this country is woefully inadequate" (Lett, 2020, para. 16) and "the lack of basic employment rights … has been ongoing for decades" (Brar, 2021, para. 3). These statements imply that the existing governmental policies determining, for example, minimum wage and other employment rights, were open for criticism prior to the COVID-19 pandemic and had already placed low-wage workers at an elevated level of risk from a social determinant perspective.

In summary, the identity of the essential worker was developed discursively. Writers of the newspaper articles used four discourse practices: including some workers and not including others to shape this representation (inclusion and exclusion), use of the interplay of texts among essential and non-essential workers (intertextuality), highlighting traits and characterizations of workers (nomination) and using text that drew on assumptions related to low wage workers and essential workers. The construction of the low-wage essential worker was developed through the discursive strategies of predominantly assumptions and representations, resulting in elevated social value being established via association with healthcare essential workers. The discursive strategy of nomination was strongly used to categorize low-wage workers as assuming increased risk in their jobs prior to the COVID-19 pandemic and increasingly so after the onset of the pandemic.

Reflections and Directions

Shifts in essential low-wage worker identity from non-essential to essential were found in this study during the COVID-19 pandemic in the articles analysed in periods two and three. For instance, societal and governmental shifts in the identity and understanding of the essential worker were found to be influenced by the discursive strategies used by the news article writers. The writers utilized the discursive strategy of nomination to highlight the positive traits of both healthcare and non-healthcare workers and to nominate both groups into the essential worker category. The implications of this shift for the future of low-wage workers, governments and employers are discussed. Perspectives on health and well-being, and a focus on occupational rights, are used to posit a more comprehensive definition of essential workers.

Implications on the Shifting Identity of the Essential Worker

Shifting from non-essential to essential identities for low-wage workers was unprecedented. Positive self-worth from low-wage earners was represented intertextually in the news articles (Sellar, 2020) when they were identified as essential. While this representation was positive, the rapid adjustment to this essential role alongside the precarious nature of their work was viewed as having a potential negative impact on worker health and well-being (Wexler et al., 2020). This finding was consistent with Park et al. (2020), who noted that low-wage workers did not assume their work would potentially put them on the front lines of a pandemic and that they would be viewed as essential workers. This change in worker identity required an atypical adjustment in their work, resulting in the potential for increased positive recognition, like health care workers, and a potential negative impact of increased exposure to health risks in the workplace. The nexus of these two elements highlights the impact on a worker's health and wellness from this shift, as having both negative and positive results.

Challenges to Occupational Rights for Low-Wage Essential Workers

The rights of all workers to participate in roles and occupations that contribute to their health and well-being are central to the definition of occupational rights (Hammell, 2008). The Government of Canada's COVID-19 response including the temporal acknowledgement of an expanded group of essential workers and resultant societal practices secondary to the COVID-19 pandemic has introduced potential challenges to occupational rights. These challenges were represented in the shift of some low-wage workers to essential work status. These challenges included reduced individual autonomy through choice (Parks et al., 2020) and the reduced ability to maintain one's health and well-being through paid work occupations with health and safety concerns and a lack of protective equipment and limited sick pay. Low-wage workers need to be empowered to advocate for the importance and meaningfulness of their paid work occupations and how these roles contribute to individual and community health and well-being. This, practically demonstrates the important consideration of occupational rights on health. This increased awareness of the value of low-wage workers and their importance in supporting individuals and communities was displayed during the COVID-19 pandemic. These experiences should challenge employers to support the attainment of occupational rights for low-wage workers.

Occupational rights are attained through what Hammell (2008) describes as participating in meaningful occupations. Productive work is a source to meet unique human physiological and psychological needs and meaningfulness through engagement in a variety of social and cultural contexts (Wilcock & Hocking, 2015). Changes in the non-essential to essential worker identity for low-wage workers may require further study of how they make sense of the work they do (being an essential worker), how they maintain their self-worth in the workplace and society (how belonging is impacted through shifts), and how they develop new competencies and confidence (in becoming an essential worker). Wilcock and Hocking (2015) outline key elements of varying roles and responsibilities, which they define as occupations. The word occupation extends beyond paid work to include other activities that people engage in and participate in. Wilcock and Hocking (2015) define being as making sense of the work they have chosen to engage in and why. The consideration of the shift from non-essential work to essential work may not allow any time for reconciliation, which may result in reduced work satisfaction and a decreased sense of personal control. Belonging reflects the people and communities that surround us through participation in occupations. Shifts to an essential worker identity can expand the scope of the community and increase connectedness to others who value the role, such as national or global groups. Becoming reflects the developmental and transformational nature of occupations and can lead to other role development. Performing work that is identified as essential may require an expansion beyond one's current capacities and strengths and may increase the demands of the role beyond initial aspirations (Wilcock & Hocking, 2015). Further examination surrounding the potential workplace health risks set against positive outcomes could advance knowledge on how to improve consistency in the well-being of low-wage workers and the attainment of occupational rights.

Occupational rights were also challenged for low-wage essential workers, specifically, including the nomination of low-wage essential workers into what Wodak (2001) described as membership in a societal out-group. A societal out-group is a group that is seen as not having access to similar levels of support or acknowledgement as other groups might enjoy. This membership in a societal out-group identified a contextual factor that negatively influenced the attainment of occupational rights for low-wage workers. Membership in this societal out-group may have further impacted access to government programmes, that is, structural factors, meant to recognize the contribution of this low-skilled group, such as the federal wage-top-up programme for minimum wage workers and other broad-based programmes rolled out during the COVID-19 pandemic, such as the Canadian Emergency Relief Benefit (CERB). CERB was an emergency relief benefit meant to provide income support to workers displaced from their workplaces secondary to COVID-19 health measures (Government of Canada, 2022). This benefit may have been inaccessible to this low-wage, low-skilled worker group for several reasons. Brar et al. (2020) in their opinion article for the Toronto Star highlighted that CERB required a level of English and internet literacy that may have disproportionately impacted low-wage, low-skilled workers secondary to their membership in racialized communities. Brar et al. (2020) further added that this federal application process may have only further perpetuated the socio-economic inequities due to these language and access barriers faced within this low-wage, low-skilled worker group.

Further negative labels were discursively used to categorize membership of low-wage essential workers as being marginalized, knowing poverty firsthand, exploited, racialized, precariously employed and socially excluded (Vohra-Miller et al., 2020). In the societal context of the COVID-19 pandemic, the oppression experienced by the low-wage essential workers was a combination of the pre-existing conditions ushered in through neoliberal governing practices that established economic inequalities specifically impacting low-wage workers (Alvarez et al., 2020; James et al., 2021). It was also underpinned by the subsequent failure of governance to ensure the safety and security of low-wage essential workers. For instance, Hanage et al. (2020) highlighted several missteps by the US government during the COVID-19 pandemic impacting low-wage workers. These findings were like the Canadian context reflected in the written news articles by Boyle and Pagliaro (2020) that included the lack of national COVID-19 workplace standards and enforcement and the lack of PPE for workplaces where low-wage workers were expected to work during COVID-19. The creation of these oppressive work conditions aligns with the position that oppression can be experienced in some social and cultural groups through the broad acceptance of societal norms and unchallenged assumptions around economic value and societal contribution in a societal context (Loustaunau et al., 2021; Northway, 1997). Oppressive working conditions for low-wage workers such as the inequities in access to proper safety protection and the expectation to continue working manifested other injustices. That of reduced autonomous participation within meaningful occupations which is foundational to occupational rights for low-wage workers. This changed for many low-wage workers who were employed in work environments with reduced health and safety oversight and mandatory access to PPE during the COVID-19 pandemic.

Specific to the examination of occupational rights, an implicit propositional assumption was utilized. Implicit propositional assumption is a discursive practice that implies being categorized as an essential worker would result in an experience of elevated social value and power in the form of commentary on government actions, as examples given by Sellar (2020). Analysis of the written texts did not demonstrate that low-wage essential workers' occupational rights were supported during the COVID-19 pandemic.

Reconsidering the Definition for Essential Workers

The Canadian government's current definition of essential services and essential workers highlights the nature of service provision being critical and not the workers themselves. The government defines an essential service as "a service, facility, or activity of the Government of Canada that is or will be, at any time, necessary for the safety or security of the public or a segment of the public" (Government of Canada, 2015, para. 5). An observation from the written news articles is that from a societal perspective, the identity of essential services was focused on the person versus the service, for example, language focused on the persons delivering the service and not the service itself. For example, the importance of grocery clerks versus grocery stores and healthcare workers versus hospitals (Benzie, 2020). These findings lay in contrast to the Government of Canada's definition of an essential service and support the need to re-frame the essential work definition, inclusive of society's prioritization of worker over work. As the authors of this chapter, we posit that the accepted definition of the essential service by the government lacks reference to the worker and that a greater focus on the worker is required to be acknowledged in times of crisis.

The research findings highlighting the shifting identity of the essential worker in this study are different than what is found in the literature, where the essentiality of the service is primary. Muñoz (2014) outlines that most governments have accepted definitions of what an essential service is, and a definition of an essential worker is lacking. The current definitions fail to address the role of the workers themselves in the delivery of these services and the impact on the health and well-being of a worker suddenly thrust into an essential role which Muñoz (2014) indicates can happen if the service is determined to be critical.

Reframing the definition to focus on the essential nature of the worker delivering critical services highlights the responsibilities of both the worker and the employer. Workers, in particular low-wage workers, must account for the potential for a change in their occupations. Acknowledging that there is a broad range of responsibilities, the role is dependent on the needs of society at a given point in time. This reframing will also support employers in acknowledging and supporting workers in developing skills and competencies in adjusting to the essential worker role and mitigating any changes to the precarious nature of their workers' employment. A revised definition will also add backing and support for decision makers to consider the needs of the workers at the forefront and move the burden off the worker to simply assume the new role with its inherent risks. For governments, institutions, employers and unions, a revised definition increases their accountability toward addressing new risks. Supporting the health of all essential workers needs to be the priority in times of societal threat. A revised definition should acknowledge that paid work occupations are culturally situated and can be influenced by a variety of factors, including changing political contexts and environments, which was the case during the COVID-19 pandemic (Wilcock & Hocking, 2015). Practically, compensation, benefits and workplace health and safety should also adopt a more fluid response in times of social crises that can return to a baseline after the disruption no longer exists. Examples of these responses include temporary increases in compensation, sick pay and vacation time.

Based on the above review of the findings of this study and the implications related to essential work, a revised definition is offered to support the reconsideration and/or the advancement and scrutiny of a new essential worker centred definition. This definition underscores the worker and accountabilities to support the worker and the service that is required in addressing social threats.

> At shifting points in time, a worker may be determined to be essential by a governing authority to preserve the physical, social, and economic safety of the public. An essential worker is one who is adequately equipped and supported by a governing authority to ensure the continuity of an essential service while supporting their identified needs related to the maintenance of the workers' health and wellbeing.

Conclusion

The shift in the identity of low-wage workers from non-essential to essential during the pandemic revealed the need to consider the health and well-being of the essential worker in times of societal and economic upheaval. The use of an occupational rights lens supports the need to consider health maintenance, including physical safety elements. Examining the meaningfulness of occupations, including paid occupations and reflecting on the implications and challenges to being, belonging and becoming as defined by Wilcock and Hocking (2015) as work identities shift from non-essential to essential is an important consideration. Informing on how best to utilize and support the essential workers in Canadian society before, during and after a crisis while minimizing undue hardships or restrictions on occupational rights will be a necessary focus of government policies or programmes aimed towards essential workers in the future.

The unique context created by the introduction of COVID-19 and our response provided an opportunity for news writers to expand the identification of those who are valued as essential workers in society for public health, political and economic reasons. The importance that the news media plays in shaping and constructing people and events was significant during the COVID-19 pandemic and should remain an active research field going forward for the learnings attained. This expanded identification brought forward new viewpoints that challenged the preponderance of the pre-COVID-19 valuing of the established front-line, first responder essential worker identity. The expanded essential worker identity affronted taken for granted, essential worker hierarchies or prioritizations and accepted definitions of essential service. The challenges to the accepted and taken-for-granted definitions, valuations and governance of essential workers offered through the pandemic response to COVID-19 further elucidated the importance of the consideration of the attainment and maintenance of occupational rights for all workers. These considerations need to be consistently upheld for workers identified as essential during a time of recognized societal need, as well as in periods of stability where their status may return to non-essential, to ensure their readiness if their work roles are required again to elevate to essential status.

References

Alvarez, C. H., Loustaunau, L., Petrucci, L., & Scott, E. (2020). Impossible choices: How workers manage unpredictable scheduling practices. *Labor Studies Journal*, *45*(2), 186–213. https://doi.org/10.1177/0160449X19835041.

Bai, Y. L., Chao-Cheng, L., Chih-Yuan, C., Jen-Yeu, C., Ching-Mo, C., & Chou, P. (2004). Survey of stress reactions among health care workers involved with the SARS outbreak. *Psychiatric Services (Washington, D.C.)*, *55*(9), 1055–1057. http://dx.doi.org/10.1176/appi.ps.55.9.1055.

Benzie, R. (8 April 2020). Ontario to increase inspections at construction sites and grocery stores to ensure workers are safe. *The Toronto Star*. https://www.thestar.com/politics/

provincial/ontario-to-increase-inspections-at-construction-sites-and-grocery-stores-to-ensure-workers-are-safe/article96f6a79b-f9f9-59f9-8905-8560e337d8e8.html.

Boyle, J., & Pagliaro, T. (30 March 2020). First homeless shelter worker tests positive for COVID-19, sparking calls for increased protection. *The Toronto Star.* https://www.thestar.com/news/gta/city-hall/first-homeless-shelter-worker-tests-positive-for-covid-19-sparking-calls-for-increased-protection/articleca4686e9-7825-5e06-a501-44a7567619d9.html.

Brar, A. (27 January 2021). Ontario continues to refuse legislation for paid sick days, says CRSB is enough. But that option is inaccessible for many. Here's the difference. *The Toronto Star.* https://www.thestar.com/opinion/contributors/ontario-continues-to-refuse-legislation-for-paid-sick-days-says-crsb-is-enough-but-that/article_889ff532-b883-5ae8-b79b-f3e1c4f83a01.html.

Canadian Public Health Association (2021). *Review of Canada's Initial Response to the COVID-19 Pandemic.* https://www.cpha.ca/review-canadas-initial-response-covid-19-pandemic.

Collins, P., Abelson, J., Pyman, H., & Lavis, J. (2006). Are we expecting too much from print media? An analysis of newspaper coverage of the 2002 Canadian healthcare reform debate. *Social Science & Medicine, 63*(1), 89–102. http://dx.doi.org/10.1016/j.socscimed.2005.12.012.

Fairclough, N., & Ebooks Corporation (2003). *Analysing Discourse: Textual Analysis for Social Research.* Routledge.

Gee, J. (2005). *An Introduction to Discourse Analysis Theory and Method* (2nd edn). Routledge. http://dx.doi.org/10.4324/9780203005675.

Gershon, R. R. M., Magda, L. A., Qureshi, K. A., Riley, H. E. M., Scanlon, E., Carney, M. T., Richards, R. J., & Sherman, M. F. (2010). Factors associated with the ability and willingness of essential workers to report to duty during a pandemic. *Journal of Occupational and Environmental Medicine, 52*(10), 995–1003. https://doi.org/10.5055/ajdm.2010.0002.

Government of Canada. (3 March 2015). *Essential Services: Frequently Asked Questions.* https://www.canada.ca/en/treasury-board-secretariat/services/labour-management/essential-services.html.

Hammell K. W., (2008). Reflections on…Well-being and occupational rights. *Canadian Journal of Occupational Therapy, 75*(1), 61–64. http://dx.doi.org/10.2182/cjot.07.007.

Hammell, K. R. W., & Beagan, B. (2017). Occupational injustice: A critique. *Canadian Journal of Occupational Therapy, 84*(1), 58–68. http://dx.doi.org/10.1177/0008417416638858.

Hanage, W., Testa, C., Chen, J., Davis, L., Pechter, E., Seminario, P., Santillana, M., & Krieger, N. (2020). COVID-19: US federal accountability for entry, spread, and inequities—Lessons for the future. *European Journal of Epidemiology, 35*(11), 995–1006. https://doi.org/10.1007/s10654-020-00689-2.

International Labour Organization (2006). *Freedom of Association: Digest of Decisions and Principles of the Freedom of Association Committee of the Governing Body of the ILO* (5th (revised) edn), https://www.ilo.org/public/libdoc/ilo/2006/106B09_305_engl.pdf.

International Labour Organization (2023). *History of the ILO.* https://www.ilo.org/global/about-the-ilo/history/lang--en/index.htm.

Institute of Labour Economics (August 2020). *Who Are the Essential Workers and Frontline Workers?* https://www.iza.org/publications/dp/13650/who-are-the-essential-and-front-line-workers.

Kari, P., Wiesner, C., Veith, S., Niilo, K., Trenz, H.-J., Dupuy, C., Van Ingelgom, V., & Liste, P. (2019). Rethinking politicisation. *Contemporary Political Theory*, *18*(2), 248–281. https://doi.org/10.1057/s41296-019-00326-y.

Kupidy, S. (2022). *A Critical Analysis of the Construction of the New Essential Worker Through the Discursive Practices of the Canadian News Media During COVID-19: Implications for Occupational Rights* [Master's thesis, Dalhousie University]. https://dalspace.library.dal.ca/items/6aed5621-22fa-4f50-b3c5-e997040872c6.

Lett, D. (2 June 2020). *Risk Payment Plan Sure to Exclude Worthy Workers.* Winnipeg Free Press. https://www.winnipegfreepress.com/local/2020/06/02/risk-payment-plan-has-value-but-worthy-workers-will-be-left-out.

Loustaunau, L., Stepick, L., Scott, E., Petrucci, L., & Henifin, M. (2021). No choice but to be essential: Expanding dimensions of precarity during COVID-19. *Sociological Perspectives*, *64*(5), 857–875. https://doi.org/10.1177/07311214211005491.

Matsuishi, K., Kawazoe, A., Imai, H., Ito, A., Mouri, K., Kitamura, N., Miyake, K., Koichi, M., Masanori, I., Takamiya, S., Hitokoto, H., & Mita, T. (2012). Psychological impact of the pandemic (H1N1) 2009 on general hospital workers in Kobe. *Psychiatry and Clinical Neurosciences*, *66*(4), 353–360. https://doi.org/10.1111/j.1440-1819.2012.02336.x.

Muñoz, C. P. (2014). Essential services, workers' freedom, and distributive justice. *Social Theory and Practice*, *40*(4), 649–672. https://doi.org/10.5840/soctheorpract201440438.

News Media Canada (2020). *Daily Newspaper Circulation Data* [Data Set]. https://nmc-mic.ca/about%20newspapers/circulation/daily-newspapers/.

Northway, R. (1997). Disability and oppression: Some implications for nurses and nursing. *Journal of Advanced Nursing*, 26(4), 736–743. https://onlinelibrary.wiley.com/doi/abs/10.1046/j.1365-2648.1997.00727.x.

Parks, C. A., Nugent, N. B., Fleischhacker, S. E., & Yaroch, A. L. (2020). Food system workers are the unexpected but under protected COVID heroes. *Journal of Nutrition*, *150*(8), 2006–2008. http://dx.doi.org/10.1093/jn/nxaa173.

Public Safety Canada (14 October 2021). *Guidance on Essential Services and Functions in Canada During the COVID-19 Pandemic.* https://www.publicsafety.gc.ca/cnt/ntnl-scrt/crtcl-nfrstrctr/esf-sfe-en.aspx.

Rafiquddin, S. (2021, October 31). Quebec's narrow asylum laws deny frontline workers resident status. *The Guardian.* https://www.theguardian.com/world/2021/oct/31/quebecs-narrow-asylum-laws-deny-frontline-workers-resident-status.

Schué, R. (15 March 2025). 'Our wings have been clipped': Quebec's 'guardian angels' in health care face deportation. *CBC News.* https://www.cbc.ca/news/canada/montreal/quebec-guardian-angels-pandemic-deportation-asylum-seekers-1.7482790.

Speer, S. (12 May 2020). Never forget the dignity of our essential workers. *National Post.* https://nationalpost.com/opinion/sean-speer-on-covid-19-never-forget-the-dignity-and-courage-of-our-essential-workers.

Tumilty, R. (18 July 2020). Are you essential? In Canada, it depends where one lives; Federal top-up pay. *National Post.* https://nationalpost.com/news/canada/are-you-an-essential-worker-in-canada-it-depends-on-where-you-live.

Vohra-Miller, S., Dosani, N., Marwaha, S., & Bulle, S. (23 December 2020). Ontario locks down on Boxing Day, but essential workers still work. Without protections like paid sick leave, it just won't work. *The Toronto Star.* https://www.thestar.com/opinion/contributors/ontario-locks-down-on-boxing-day-but-essential-workers-still-work-without-protections-like-paid/article_af932c55-6c57-58a7-b3ee-cac951530a90.html.

Wexler, S., Engel, R. J., Steiner, E., & Petracchi, H. (2020). "It is truly a struggle to survive": The hardships of living on low wages. *Families in Society*, *101*(3), 275–288. https://doi.org/10.1177/1044389420928270.

WFP Editorial Board (13 May 2020). *No Serenade, But Wage Hike Is Warranted.* Winnipeg Free Press. https://www.winnipegfreepress.com/opinion/editorials/2020/05/13/no-serenade-but-wage-hike-is-warranted.

Wilcock, A., & Hocking, C. (2015). *An Occupational Perspective of Health* (3rd ed.). SLACK Inc.

Williams, J. C., Anderson, N., Holloway, T., Samford III, E., Eugene, J., & Isom, J. (2020). Reopening the United States: Black and Hispanic workers are essential and expendable again. *American Journal of Public Health*, *110*(10), 1506–1508. http://dx.doi.org/10.2105/AJPH.2020.305879.

Wodak, R., & Meyer, M. (2001). *Methods of Critical Discourse Analysis* (1st ed.). SAGE Publications Ltd. http://dx.doi.org/10.4135/9780857028020.

Wong, E. L., Wong, S. Y., Lee, N., Cheung, A., & Griffiths, S. (2012). Healthcare workers' duty concerns of working in the isolation ward during the novel H1N1 pandemic. *Journal of Clinical Nursing*, *21*(9–10), 1466–1475. http://dx.doi.org/10.1111/j.1365-2702.2011.03783.x.

NOTES ON CONTRIBUTORS

ROKSANA (ROXY) DOBRIN-DE GRACE is a PhD candidate in Psychological Science at Toronto Metropolitan University in the Early Childhood Cognition Lab. Her research focuses on examining the development of prosocial behaviours in early childhood, particularly politeness and considerate behaviour, in experimental laboratory settings.

ELIZABETH KAY-RAINING BIRD, Professor Emeritus in the School of Communication Sciences and Disorders at Dalhousie University, is a researcher of language development in culturally and linguistically diverse children with language-learning difficulties. She also advocates for basic income as a poverty elimination and health promotion strategy.

DIANA BURCHELL is a Research Project Manager in Research and Assessment Services at the York Region District School Board. She is passionate about investigating and improving the accessibility of our education system for multilingual students and students with disabilities.

KATHLEEN HIPFNER-BOUCHER is a Senior Research Officer in the Multilingualism and Literacy Lab at the Ontario Institute for Studies in Education.

Her research interests include the oral language skills that support reading among bi- and multilingual children and early literacy screening.

Xi Chen is Professor at the Ontario Institute for Studies in Education. Her research specializes in language and literacy development of bilingual children. She examines theoretical models of literacy development, cross-language transfer, dyslexia and reading comprehension difficulties among bilingual children.

Serenity Friskie (she/they) is an Equity and Engagement Specialist at Foundry BC, a researcher at SARAVYC, and an Indigenous wellness educator. Of mixed European and Indigenous ancestry, they advocate for justice, youth mental health, culturally safe care and community spaces on unceded Coast Salish territories.

Sunny Manhas, MSW, (she/they) is a settler on the continually occupied territories and ancestral lands of the Skwxwú7mesh-ulh Temíx̱w (Squamish), xʷməθkʷəy̓əm (Musqueam) and səl̓ilwətaʔɬ təməxʷ (Tsleil-Waututh), and a healthcare social worker practising in Vancouver's Downtown Eastside.

Zineb Boudiba is a Doctor of Philosophy, research fellow, and sessional lecturer at Canterbury Christ Church University. Her research explores resilience and professional identity among special education teachers, focusing on systemic challenges. She teaches various modules and is committed to improving educational practices and supporting teachers in diverse contexts.

Steven Kupidy is a Clinical Occupational Therapist with 25+ years of experience, currently focusing on expanding Occupational Therapy access in rural communities through innovation. His expertise spans clinical care and healthcare leadership, with a passion for promoting the role of occupation in well-being and work.

Lynn Shaw is Professor and Director of the School of Occupational Therapy at Western University. She is an occupational scientist focused on equitable work transitions, mobility, and addressing work disparities for groups of workers. She is also President of the Canadian Society for Occupational Science.

FSC
www.fsc.org
MIX
Papier | Fördert gute Waldnutzung
FSC® C083411

Kolibri 360 GmbH
Ferdinand-Jühlke-Straße 7
99095 Erfurt, Deutschland
produktsicherheit@kolibri360.de

Druck:
CPI Druckdienstleistungen GmbH
im Auftrag der
Kolibri 360 GmbH
Ferdinand-Jühlke-Str. 7
99095 Erfurt